HELP!

The Quick Guide to First Aid for Your Dog

HELP!

The Quick Guide to First Aid for Your Dog

Michelle Bamberger, D.V.M.

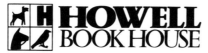

HOWELL BOOK HOUSE

New York

Maxwell Macmillan Canada
Toronto

Maxwell Macmillan International
New York   Oxford   Singapore   Sydney

Howell Book House
Macmillan Publishing Company
866 Third Avenue
New York, NY 10022

Maxwell Macmillan Canada, Inc.
1200 Eglinton Avenue East
Suite 200
Don Mills, Ontario M3C 3N1

Macmillan Publishing Company is part of the Maxwell Communication Group of Companies.

Library of Congress Cataloging-in-Publication Data
Bamberger, Michelle.
  Help!: the quick guide to first aid for your dog/Michelle
Bamberger.
    p.   cm.
  Includes bibliographical references (p. 137).
  ISBN 0-87605-557-9
  1. Dogs—Wounds and injuries—Treatment. 2. Dogs—Diseases—
Treatment. 3. First aid for animals. I. Title. II. Title: Quick
guide to first aid for your dog.
      SF991.B28   1993
  636.7′08960252—dc20   92-33692
                CIP

Macmillan books are available at special discounts for bulk purchases for sales promotions, premiums, fund-raising, or educational use. For details, contact:

Special Sales Director
Macmillan Publishing Company
866 Third Avenue
New York, NY 10022

10 9 8 7 6 5 4 3 2 1

Printed in the United States of America

Contents

Acknowledgments

THIS BOOK would not have been possible without the help of many human and canine friends. My editor at Howell Book House, Marcy Zingler, has shown great enthusiasm for this book from the very beginning and continues to do so. Dr. Susan Begg and Dr. Sarah King kindly took time away from their own small animal practices to read through an initial draft of this book and make helpful comments and suggestions. For having helped make all the illustrations in this book possible, I thank several owners and their dogs: Margaret and Norman Velykis with Tasha and Schnippy, Denny and Zelda Johnston with Alexis and Michael and Myrna Schoenfeld with Katie. For help with design concepts, I thank Dr. Nena Winand and Dr. Martina Altshul with Turbo. I heartily thank fellow writer and friend, Bryna Fireside, for encouragement and valuable advice. I am indebted to my parents, Joseph and Helen Bamberger, for watching my son Benjamin so that I could meet the deadline for this book. Finally, I am most grateful to Professor Robert Oswald for invaluable editorial comments and for entertaining our son so that I could write this book.

Michelle Bamberger, D.V.M.
Ithaca, New York

HELP!

The Quick Guide to First Aid for Your Dog

Introduction

THIS BOOK is written for dog owners who want to know how to act responsibly in an emergency. It is not meant to replace veterinarians; rather, it attempts to make dog owners more aware of how to approach emergencies and how to handle them effectively until a veterinarian can be reached.

I have taught first aid to pet owners, SPCA personnel and animal health technicians. Since I have been unable to recommend a book which specifically covers emergency care in any easy-to-understand yet thorough manner, I decided to write and illustrate one. This book is an outgrowth of my course and contains many of the illustrations I used to describe first aid techniques to my students.

I recommend that rather than "spot reading," readers begin with the first two chapters. Together these chapters describe a general approach which can be used in all emergencies. In addition, Chapter 1 describes basic life saving techniques, while Chapter 2 lists first aid for specific conditions you might find while examining your dog.

Typical emergencies are discussed in Chapter 3. **Don't wait until the emergency occurs to read this chapter.** Acquaint yourself with the signs and first aid for each emergency so that if one does occur, you will be able to recognize it and will have an idea of what steps to take. Wound and fracture care are described in Chapter 4. In this chapter, bandages for different parts of the body are illustrated in a step-by-step fashion. Finally, Chapter 5 gives you a chance to encounter some real-life emergencies and allows you to decide what to do (the answers are in Appendix 3).

First Aid Supplies

THE FOLLOWING is a list of first aid supplies that you
should have available in your home:

Adhesive tape
Blankets
Board or window screen
Bucket
Cardboard boxes
Cotton balls
Cotton roll
Cotton swabs
Cup
Gauze roll
Magazines
Masking tape
Medications (see Appendix 2 for use and dosages)
   Antibiotic ointment (Neosporin® or Bacitracin)
   Aspirin (buffered or enteric coated)
   Activated charcoal
   Hydrogen peroxide (3%)
   Syrup of ipecac
   Vegetable or mineral oil
Medicine dropper

Newspapers
Pads (preferably nonstick)
Pencil
Scissors
Sheets (bed)
Soap
Thermometer (preferably digital)
Towels
Tweezers
Washcloth

1

What to Do First: Basic Life Saving Techniques

IF YOU FOUND your dog injured and unable to move, would you know what to do first? In an emergency such as this, your dog may be suffering from more than one type of injury.

For instance, if the dog had been hit by a car, you might notice several problems right away: a large bleeding wound over his back and a fractured hind leg. On further exam, you discover your dog is in shock and probably has internal injuries. Your knowledge of what to do first and use of standard first aid techniques will dramatically affect the dog's recovery.

In this chapter, we will discuss the basic steps used to approach all emergencies and the first aid methods for the most life threatening situations. Section 1 will cover **triage**, which is the art of determining the problems and then sorting them according to severity. Section 2 will discuss **restraint and transport**; these techniques are often necessary before any first aid can be given. Sections 3 through 6 will be used to explain and illustrate first aid methods used to treat **extreme emergency conditions:** *cardiopulmonary failure, drowning, choking, shock and severe bleeding.*

Whatever the emergency, having your dog evaluated by your veterinarian is critical. You may administer first aid while on the way to the veterinarian. Alternatively, you may bring your dog in for a checkup after the dog is stabilized. Even if you feel your dog has completely recovered, you should still call your veterinarian and describe the emergency. The veterinarian may be able to give you advice and suggestions to help your dog make an even quicker recovery. Remember to always call ahead before bringing your dog to an emergency clinic or veterinary hospital.

SECTION 1: TRIAGE

Assessing Your Dog

Before taking any action in an emergency, **make sure the environment is safe**. You will have to move your dog to a safer location before doing anything else, if the emergency takes place on a busy road, in a burning building or near electrical hazards. If your dog is uncooperative, you may have to use a muzzle or provide some other form of restraint before you can start first aid (see Restraint and Transport, Section 2). Figure 1-1 illustrates a general approach which can be used in all situations.

Once the environment is safe for you and your dog, your next step is to assess your dog's condition quickly, and **make a mental list of the major problems.**

Once you have a good idea of the injuries your dog has suffered, you can **rank these problems from most severe to least severe.** This two-step process is called *triage* and should always be carried out before any first aid is administered. It assures that you will be concentrating your efforts where they are needed most and increasing the chances that your dog will survive.

On approaching your dog in an emergency, you may see some obvious problems. However, other problems may be present and possibly be even more life threatening. Fortunately, you can quickly evaluate your dog by using a few simple procedures (see Figure 1-1).

1. First, check to see if the dog is responsive. You can do this by calling your dog's name, clapping your hands or gently tapping the dog's head. Your dog should move and may bark or come to you.
2. If the dog does not respond in any way, you should immediately check the airway, breathing and circulation.
3. If necessary, start cardiopulmonary resuscitation (see Section 3 and Figure 1-14).

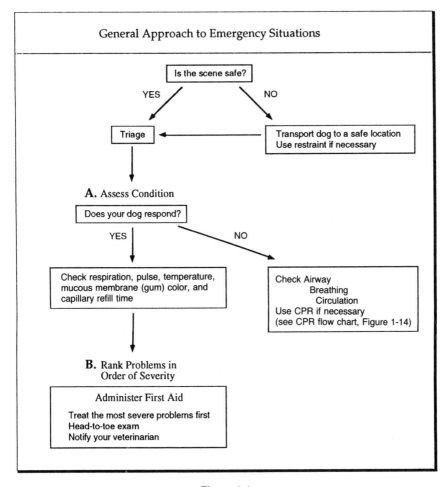

Figure 1-1

Respiration Rate

If your dog does respond, the next step is to take a respiration rate (breaths/minute; see Figure 1-2). Although **normal rates of respiration are 10 to 30 breaths/minute,** dogs may pant up to 200 breaths/minute. A *decreased respiration rate* may result from poisoning, hypothermia or the late stages of shock. An *increased rate* may be caused by excitement, heat, exercise, pain or the early stages of shock.

Pulse

Once you have determined the respiration rate, it is time to take the pulse (beats/minute; see Figure 1-3 [Top left]). If you can't feel a pulse

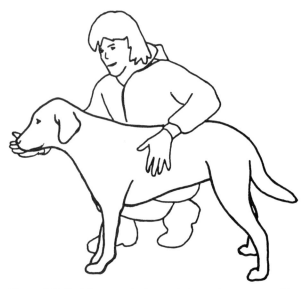

Figure 1-2: To take your dog's respiratory rate, you can either place one hand on the rib cage and feel for the chest moving in and out or you can place your hand in front of your dog's nostrils, feeling for air movement. Either way, you should count the breaths for 15 seconds and then multiply by 4 to get the number of breaths per minute.

in this location, feel for the heartbeat (see Figure 1-3 [Top right and Bottom]). **The normal pulse rate is between 60 to 120 beats/minute**. Large or athletic dogs tend to be at the lower end of the scale while small dogs and puppies are usually at the upper end. In the late stages of shock and in cases of hypothermia, the pulse may be less than 60 beats/minute. On the other hand, excitement, fever, heart failure, electric shock, snake bite, poisonings, severe pain and the early stages of shock may result in a pulse that is higher than normal.

Temperature

After getting the pulse and respiration rates, take your dog's temperature. You may have to muzzle the dog (see Section 2) in order to do this even if the dog's temperature has been taken many times before. You can make it less uncomfortable by using a small amount of water soluble jelly, such as K-Y®, on the tip of the thermometer. Insert the thermometer into the rectum approximately 1 inch. It is best to use *a digital thermome-*

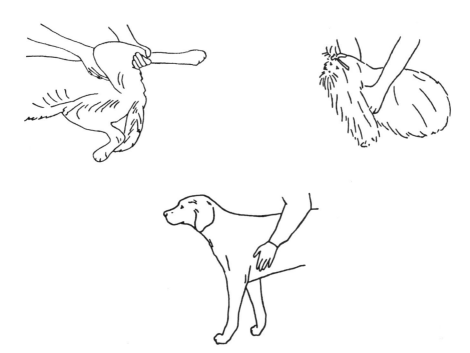

Figure 1-3: Top left: To take your dog's pulse rate, place the tips of your fingers along the inside of the thigh, in the groin area, and feel for a pulse. The pulse will arise from a large blood vessel called the femoral artery. Do not press down too hard as you will not be able to feel the pulse. Count the pulse for 15 seconds and then multiply by 4 to get the beats per minute. **Top right:** To feel the heartbeat in a small dog, place your hand on the left side of the rib cage, about 1 inch behind the point of the elbow. Count the beats for 15 seconds and then multiply by 4 to get the beats per minute. **Bottom:** To feel the heartbeat in a large dog, place your hand on the left side of the rib cage, about 2 to 3 inches behind the point of the elbow. Count the beats for 15 seconds and then multiply by 4 to get the beats per minute.

ter, as these are very accurate and can be read *within 1.5 minutes.* If you must use *a glass thermometer,* remember to *wait 3 minutes* before reading the temperature. The **normal temperature** range for a dog **is 101.5°F to 102.5°F.** Temperatures above normal are commonly due to nervousness, heat, exercise or infection. Temperatures of only 1 to 2 degrees above normal may be treated with buffered or enteric coated aspirin (see Appendix 2 for dosage).

If a low-grade fever such as this persists for more than a few days or is accompanied by other signs (such as vomiting, diarrhea, convulsions), you should call your veterinarian. Temperatures below normal result mostly from exposure to cold weather for long periods or to severe shock. Temperature extremes and their treatments are discussed in Chapter 3, Section 11.

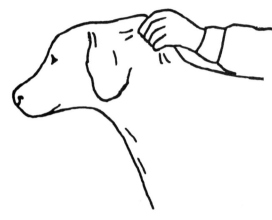

Figure 1-4: To determine if a dog is dehydrated, pick up the skin along the back of your dog's neck with your thumb and forefinger. Then let it go. It should go back down immediately. If the skin does not go back down immediately, then your dog is dehydrated. The longer it takes to go down, the more dehydrated your dog is.

Dehydration

While you are taking the temperature, you can check to see if your dog is dehydrated by using the technique described in Figure 1-4. If you still are not sure whether or not your dog is dehydrated, you can also check to see if the gums are tacky or dry to the touch of your fingertips (see Figure 1-5). **Normally, the gums will feel quite wet.** Tackiness indicates dehydration. Dehydration commonly occurs with shock and prolonged vomiting and diarrhea.

It is important to know that old dogs may appear dehydrated when they are really not because skin elasticity decreases with age, while overweight dogs may appear to be hydrated even when they are really not, because fat increases skin elasticity. In cases such as these, be sure to check the gums.

Circulation—Gums and Capillary Refill Time

In addition to taking the pulse, you can use two simple procedures to check the circulatory system:

1. Look at the color of the gums.
2. Check the capillary refill time, also via the gums.

As shown in Figure 1-5 [Left], put your hand on your dog's muzzle and use your thumb to lift your dog's lip up enough to expose the gums. First examine the color. **Normally the gums are pale pink.**

If they are very pale to *white* in color, your dog may be in shock or may be anemic due to fleas, ticks or worms. If the gums are *blue,* this may indicate shock, heart failure, lung failure or poisoning. *Red,* con-

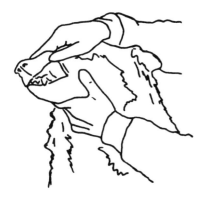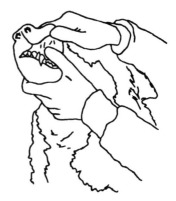

Figure 1-5: Left: To expose your dog's gums, put one hand on the top of your dog's muzzle, lifting up the lip. The other hand cups the lower muzzle for restraint. This is a good position to look at the color of the gums, take the capillary refill time and check the gums for tackiness (dehydration). **Right:** To take the capillary refill time, one hand rests on the upper muzzle, with the thumb pulling the lip up. The second hand rests under the muzzle. Use the thumb of this hand to press firmly on the gums, then immediately remove your thumb. The blanched area should return to a normal pink color within 2 seconds.

gested gums may mean your dog either has an abdominal emergency, has been poisoned by carbon monoxide or has severe heart/lung failure. If the gums are *yellow*, your dog may have liver failure. If you aren't quite sure of the yellow color, check the color under your dog's tongue or the white of the eye. Check the gums for small red spots. These are pinpoint hemorrhages and are a signal that your dog has a bleeding problem.

After you have had a good look at the color of the gums, take the capillary refill time. This is the time it takes for the capillaries, which are the tiny blood vessels just under the gums and skin, to refill once they have been emptied by manual pressure. To perform this procedure, see Figure 1-5 [Right]. If the color takes longer than 2 seconds to return, your dog has poor circulation. **Normal capillary refill time is under 2 seconds.**

Ranking the Problems

After taking the temperature, pulse and respiration and evaluating the hydration status and circulatory system, you will have a good idea of the general condition of your dog. While each emergency situation will produce a different set of problems, the method for ranking the most life threatening situations will remain the same.

At the top of the list are situations where your dog is not responsive: no pulse and no breathing or no breathing and a pulse. Both conditions are dire and require knowledge of a cardiopulmonary resuscitation technique (see Section 3).

Drowning is a good example of an emergency which may produce either one of these conditions. In drowning, the lungs fill up with water and breathing is impossible. Drowning is discussed in Section 4 of this chapter.

Choking is next on the list because your dog will not get the normal amount of oxygen into the lungs. If not helped immediately (see Section 5), the dog could lose consciousness and stop breathing.

Shock and severe bleeding are listed next. Shock is an insidious condition which accompanies many emergencies, and without intervention, the heart and lungs will stop functioning and your dog will have to be resuscitated. Severe bleeding is a major cause of shock; both are discussed in Section 6.

You may be faced with many other emergencies such as poisonings, burns and allergic reactions, which may seem just as life threatening as the conditions discussed above. These emergencies are not discussed here for triage purposes because their ranking is so highly dependent upon each individual emergency. For instance, a poisoning may or may not be life threatening depending upon the poisoning agent, how much was taken, the age of the dog, the time which elapses until first aid is given and other conditions which develop as a result of the poisoning (shock), etc. These emergencies are discussed in Chapter 3.

Summary

The following example illustrates how to use triage in a typical emergency situation:

> You come home to find your dog on your front lawn, seemingly asleep. You call, but your dog does not respond. As you approach your dog, you notice a bloody wound on the back of the dog's leg. You evaluate your dog and find there is a pulse but no breathing.
>
> In a case such as this, it is important to remember that *you must resuscitate your dog before tending to the wound*. It is tempting to want to take a few minutes to apply a bandage, but in that time you will lose precious moments which could have been spent trying to resuscitate your dog. However, in a situation where two people are present to help, one would get started on resuscitation while the other could quickly apply a bandage and then assist with the resuscitation.

In order to respond effectively to an emergency, you should follow the steps listed below before administering first aid:

Assess the environment

- Is it safe?
- Does your dog need restraint?
- Does your dog need to be transported immediately?

Triage

Assess your dog's condition

- Respiration
- Pulse
- Temperature
- Hydration status
- Gum color
- Capillary refill time

Rank the problems from most severe to least severe

- No breathing, no pulse
- No breathing, pulse
- Choking
- Shock/severe bleeding

SECTION 2: RESTRAINT AND TRANSPORT

Sometimes emergencies occur in locations which are too dangerous for you to perform even a quick evaluation of your dog, much less administer first aid. If your dog is hit by a car in the middle of a busy road, your first priority must be to move your dog to a safe location. During the move, restraint is necessary so that you or anyone helping you doesn't get bitten and proper transport is required so that severe injuries are not exacerbated. This chapter will explain and illustrate easily applied methods for effective restraint and safe transport.

Restraint

The degree of restraint varies with the type of emergency, the size and behavior of your dog and the presence or absence of another person to help. In general, you should use the least amount of restraint necessary for a situation, because more restraint will make you tire faster and may make your dog less willing to cooperate. You should also constantly reassure your dog in a calm, gentle voice during the entire procedure.

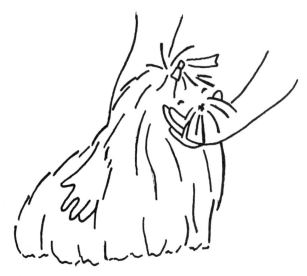

Figure 1-6: To hold a small dog, place one hand under your dog's muzzle so that your thumb is on one side and the rest of your fingers are on the other side. Make sure your grip is not so tight that breathing or circulation is restricted. If you are by yourself, your other hand is then free to perform first aid or examine your dog. With help, you can place your other hand over your dog's hip for a more secure hold.

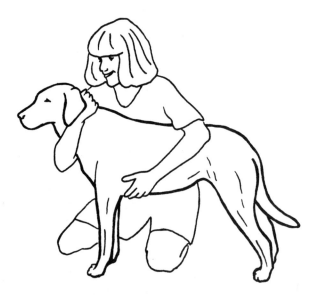

Figure 1-7: To hold a large dog, wrap your arm around the front of your dog's neck and as far around the back of the neck as possible. This leaves your other arm free to examine your dog or give first aid.

Restraining Your Dog Without Assistance

If you are by yourself and you have a small dog, you should use the hold shown in Figure 1-6. This hold will allow you to keep your dog's head and neck in control while using your free hand to perform first aid. With a large dog in the same situation, the hold shown in Figure 1-7 will give you the same control as in Figure 1-6, again freeing your other hand.

Any hold on any size dog will be difficult if that dog is biting. If you have a dog who tends to bite, you should muzzle your dog before proceeding any further. But if your dog doesn't usually bite when frightened or hurt, you should avoid using a muzzle. The muzzle will upset your dog unnecessarily when a good hold would have done just fine.

If you do decide to muzzle your dog, you won't need another person to assist you as this is something you can do yourself. What you will need are strips of soft, strong material such as bed sheet or gauze bandage wrap. The strips should be 2 to 3 feet long and be 2 to 3 inches wide. *Do*

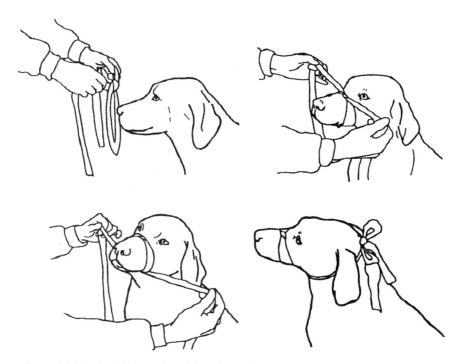

Figure 1-8: Top left: Using a 2- to 3-foot piece of cloth, make an overhand loop leaving a large enough space for your dog's muzzle. **Top right:** Quickly slip this over your dog's muzzle and tie it down firmly on top without making a knot. **Bottom left:** Quickly cross the bandage ends of the cloth underneath the dog's chin. **Bottom right:** Bring both ends up behind your dog's ears and tie a bow knot securely.

not use rope, chain, twine or any material which may cut or inflame the skin when tightened.

The secret to *muzzling* your dog is to *be fast*. Putting on a muzzle is much safer with a longer piece of material because you can tie the overhand loop before it goes on your dog (see Figure 1-8). This muzzle must be tied firmly to be effective; as long as the muzzling material is soft, do not be afraid to tie down tightly.

If you have only a short piece of material available for a muzzle, for instance a kerchief, see Figure 1-9. This method should only be used as a last resort for two reasons. First, your hands are so close to your dog's mouth when you tie the overhand loop that you will risk getting bitten. Second, because this muzzle is not secured behind the ears (compare Figures 1-8 and 1-9), your dog may be able to loosen it so much that the muzzle might come off.

If you don't want to use a cloth tie to muzzle your dog and you don't want to get bitten, then you should invest in a nylon muzzle (see Figure 1-10). These muzzles may be more effective than a tie muzzle but a little harder to put on a biting dog, as your hands will be close to your dog's mouth as you fit the muzzle over the dog's face. Whichever method

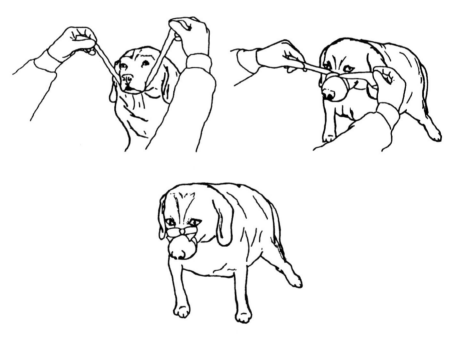

Figure 1-9: Top left: If only a short piece of material is available, hold the ends to both sides of your dog's head with the middle of the material under your dog's chin. **Top right:** Quickly tie an overhand loop and tighten down. **Bottom:** To secure the muzzle, tie a bow knot.

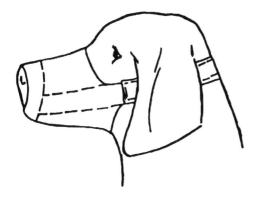

Figure 1-10: Nylon dog muzzle made to the shape of a dog's head. Fit over your dog's face quickly and carefully.

you choose, remember that a muzzle should not be used if your dog is having breathing difficulties, is vomiting or has severe head, mouth or abdominal injuries. Also the muzzle should be removed as soon as possible because eating, drinking and panting are impossible while the muzzle is on your dog. After your dog is muzzled, you can hold as in Figure 1-6 for a small dog, or Figure 1-7 for a large dog. Both holds will still allow you to have a free hand to perform first aid.

Restraining Your Dog with Assistance

If an emergency occurs while bystanders are present, enlist their help. Your dog will be held more securely and first aid will go faster. For a small dog, use the hold shown in Figure 1-6 but this time put your left hand over your dog's left hip and hold the dog close to your body. If you have a large dog, hold as shown in Figure 1-11. Remember to reassure your dog while first aid is being given.

Even if you have help, you should still use a muzzle if your dog is biting or has a tendency to bite. Not only will the muzzle protect you, but also anybody who decides to help you. Once the muzzle is in place, one person will hold using the method shown in Figure 1-6 for a small dog or Figure 1-11 for a large dog. The other person will then give first aid.

TRANSPORT

How you choose to move your dog will largely depend on whether or not there are any broken bones. If your dog has suffered any severe head, neck, back or leg injuries, such as falling from a high place or being hit by a car, then there is a good chance that there will be fractures

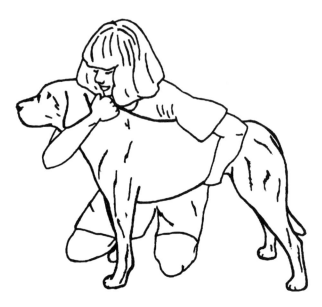

Figure 1-11: To hold a large dog when another person is present who can help you, follow the same procedure as in Figure 1-7, but now wrap your other arm under the dog's abdomen in a gentle hug.

in the spinal column, pelvis and/or legs (see Chapter 4, Section 3). In these situations, you must transport your dog properly if you want to avoid causing further injury and pain.

Transporting a Dog with Spinal Cord Injury

The signs of a spinal cord injury include: unconsciousness; blood or clear fluid from the ear, nose or mouth; pupils of different sizes; shock and paralysis.

Without Assistance: Which method you choose for transport will also depend on the size of your dog, what materials you have available and whether or not you have assistance. There are a few methods you can use if you are by yourself and you want to move a dog showing signs of spinal cord damage.

For a small dog, the method of choice is to use a firm surface, such as a plywood board, window screen or flat sled. Gently ease your dog onto this surface, which ideally is a little bigger than your dog and will fit into your car (see Figure 1-12 [Left]). In general, you should always lay the dog on its side, but if your dog seems uncomfortable in this

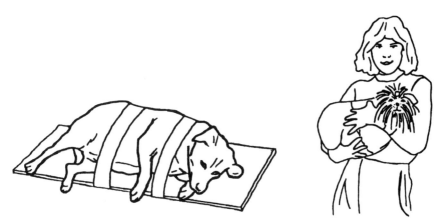

Figure 1-12: Left: To transport a dog with suspected spinal cord injury, use a plywood board or another firm, flat surface. Gently ease your dog onto the board without twisting or bending his body. Loosely tie your dog to the board with cloth to keep him from falling off. **Right:** To transport a small dog with suspected spinal cord injury when no firm surface is available, ease your dog onto a blanket and gently wrap the blanket around him, taking care not to bend or twist his body. Carry your dog in your arms, keeping the back as straight as possible by supporting the front and hind ends.

position, a prone position (on the chest) is satisfactory. *It is extremely important not to bend or twist your dog during the move.* The second method uses a large towel or blanket, see Figure 1-12 [Right].

Using the same principle of supporting the back, you can move a large dog with spinal cord injury by yourself as shown in Figure 1-13.

With Assistance: If you have assistance, transporting a dog with spinal cord damage is much less difficult than doing it by yourself. For any size dog, the best method is to use a firm surface as described above (see Figure 1-12 [Left]). If one is not available, gently ease your dog onto a blanket or large towel and have each person hold a corner of the blanket. Move both dog and blanket by holding the four corners very tightly, to give good support.

With or without help, you should keep the concept of support in mind when transporting a dog with spinal cord injuries in your car. Whether you use a box, carrier or the backseat itself, remember to support the body fully as you pick up and put down your dog.

If there is no one who can sit in the backseat to keep your dog from moving around as you drive, place pillows or rolled towels to either side of the box, carrier or the dog on the backseat. You should also put some pillows between the front seat and the backseat so that your dog doesn't fall off the seat at a sudden stop.

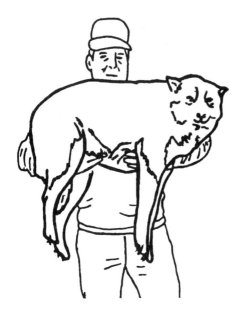

Figure 1-13: To transport a medium to large dog with suspected spinal cord injury when no firm surface is available, carry your dog by putting one arm between the front legs and one arm between the hind legs. Your hands should now be pointing toward each other under your dog's abdomen. Lean your dog's body toward your body, keeping the dog's back as straight as possible by supporting both the front and hind ends.

Transporting a Dog with Leg or Pelvic Fractures

The signs of leg fractures include: soreness, swelling, and limping.

Dogs with leg or pelvic fractures should also be carefully transported. To move a dog showing signs of leg fractures, first apply a temporary splint to the broken leg (see Figures 4-18 and 4-19 and Chapter 4, Section 3). The splint will greatly decrease the swelling which accompanies fractures and make it much easier to repair later. The splint may also allow your dog to stand, if there is only the one fracture.

If your dog can walk with the splint, you can allow it.

If not, assume that the dog may also have a spinal cord injury or other fractures of which you are unaware. In this case, follow one of the methods shown in Figures 1-12 and 1-13, depending on the size of your dog, availability of materials and presence of help.

Signs of pelvic fractures include the inability to move the back legs, or once standing, the back legs go out sideways.

To move a dog exhibiting these signs you should follow one of the methods shown in Figures 1-12 and 1-13. If your dog wants to stand, first apply adhesive tape hobbles (see Figure 4-17 and Chapter 4, Section 3).

Transporting an Ambulatory Dog

All dogs, including those that can walk, need to be restrained in the car for safety purposes. For small dogs, use a pet carrier. If you do not have a carrier, then use a blanket (see Figure 1-12 [Right]), a box with several holes in the top, pillowcase or your own coat sleeve. To transport a medium to large size dog in a car without a carrier, try to get someone to sit in the backseat with the dog until you arrive at the hospital. Be sure to call the hospital before leaving so they can be expecting you.

Whatever injuries have been sustained, during transport you should keep the dog warm and watch out for **the initial signs of shock: pale gums, restlessness, a rapid, weak pulse and an increased breathing rate**. Unfortunately, shock may occur while you are transporting your dog to the hospital. For more on shock, see Section 6.

In summary, knowledge of proper restraint and transport techniques is of great importance in trying to help a sick or injured dog. With or without assistance, you have a number of effective methods from which to choose depending upon the circumstances of the injury and the availability of materials.

SECTION 3: Cardiopulmonary Resuscitation (CPR)

Cardiopulmonary resuscitation is a powerful technique: it provides much-needed oxygen to the brain, heart and other organs during the time when the heart has stopped and your dog cannot breathe independently. Through your efforts, you may resuscitate the dog yourself or at least enable a veterinarian to take over and use more advanced CPR techniques to save your dog.

As mentioned in the triage section, the first step in assessing a dog's condition is to determine if there is any response to your voice or touch. If your dog does respond, you should evaluate his condition and determine which problem needs to be treated first (see Section 1). However, if there is no response, you must assume that you may have to resuscitate the dog and begin the mechanics of CPR technique immediately, as discussed below. If someone is around who can drive, remember that this technique can be used in the car. This would give your dog the best chance of survival, since you have started resuscitation immediately and are on your way to an emergency clinic or veterinary hospital.

The **technique of CPR** will be discussed by the use of a flow chart

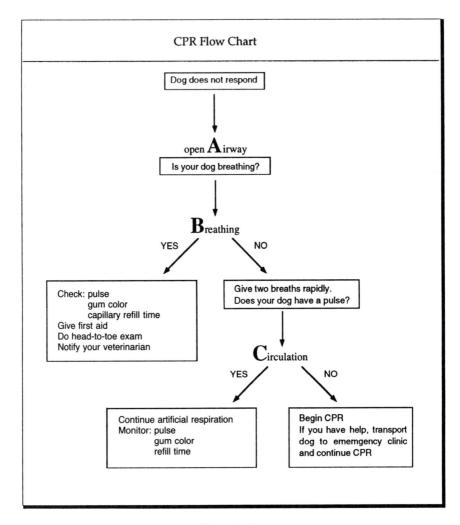

Figure 1-14

(see Figure 1-14) which **incorporates the three basic concepts of** *airway, breathing and circulation*. Beginning on the flow chart where your dog is not responsive, the *first step* must be to *open an airway* (see Figure 1-15).

Next you will *determine if your dog is breathing* (see Figure 1-16). You will be looking at the chest to see if there is any rising or falling and you will be listening and feeling for air movement against your cheek. If your dog is breathing, you should note the rate.

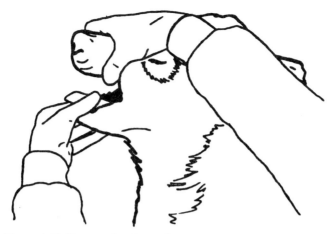

Figure 1-15: To open the airway, first extend the head and neck. Put one hand on the top of the muzzle to open the mouth and grab the end of the tongue with your free hand and pull it forward. If you cannot get a good grip on the tongue with your bare fingers, try grabbing the tongue with a cloth. Clear the mouth of all food, vomit, etc.

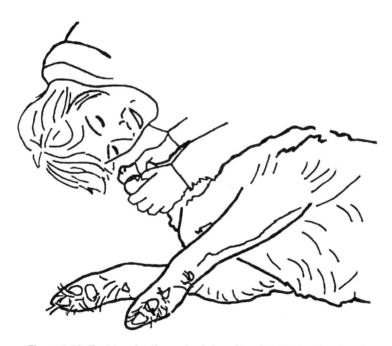

Figure 1-16: To determine if your dog is breathing, hold the head and neck extended and tongue rolled forward. Bend down close to your dog, with your face turned toward his chest and your cheek close to his mouth and nose. Look, listen and feel for breathing for 10 seconds.

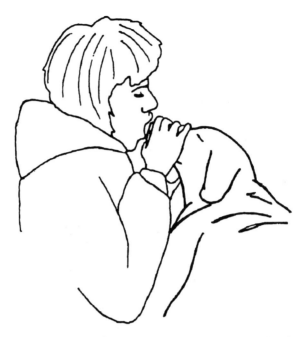

Figure 1-17: To give artificial respiration, have the head and neck extended, the tongue rolled forward and the mouth closed shut by holding both of your hands around your dog's muzzle. Place your mouth over your dog's nose and blow air into your dog's nostrils.

Then take the pulse and temperature, and check the color, refill time and hydration status (see Section 1). You should notify your veterinarian immediately and continue to monitor the above parameters.

If your dog is not breathing, you must begin artificial respiration (see Figure 1-17). You should see your dog's chest expand. Then take your mouth away so that air can leave the lungs. You may not see his chest expand for three reasons. First, you may not be holding the dog's mouth and lips tightly closed. Second, you may not be blowing with enough force to make the lungs expand. And third, your dog may have an obstruction in the lower airway. Unless you have witnessed your dog choking on an object before he became nonresponsive, you should assume that the chest didn't expand for either of the first two reasons. Whether you have seen your dog's chest expand or not, next *give 2 more breaths quickly.*

Circulation is checked next by taking your dog's pulse or heartbeat for 10 seconds (see Figure 1-3). If you do find that your dog *does have a pulse,* but is *not breathing,* you must continue artificial respiration. If

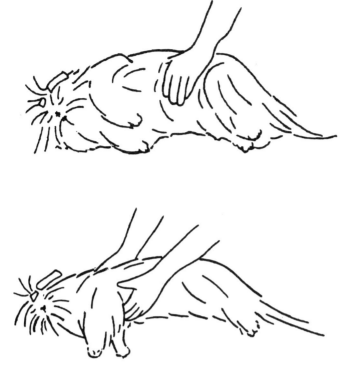

Figure 1-18: Top: To remove air from the stomach, place the flat of your hand on the left side of your dog, just behind the ribs, and push down gently. **Bottom:** To compress the chest of a small dog, open your hand around the widest part of the chest and within 1 inch of the point of the elbow so that your thumb is on one side and the rest of your fingers are on the other side. Depress the rib cage from both sides 1 to 1.5 inches at a rate of 120 to 150 times per minute.

you have *a small dog* (less than 25 pounds), you should continue the breaths at *20–25 times per minute (1 breath every 3 seconds)*. For a *medium to large dog,* the rate is *15 to 20 times per minute (1 breath every 4 seconds)*. Your breaths should be slow and last 1 to 1.5 seconds each. After a minute's worth of artificial respiration, take the pulse for 5 seconds and then look, listen and feel to see if breathing has returned for 5 seconds. If breathing has not returned, continue artificial respiration, stopping every minute to monitor the pulse and breathing.

Sometimes, air collects in the stomach and this can be removed by pushing down with the flat of your hand on the left side, just behind the ribs (see Figure 1-18 [Top]; NOTE: This is most effective in smaller dogs). You should do this every few minutes or so. If breathing does come back,

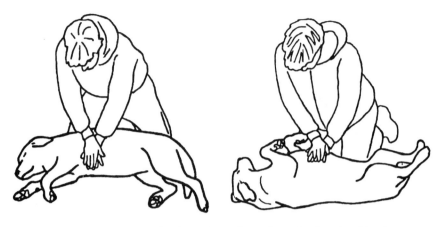

Figure 1-19: Left: To compress the chest of a medium to large dog from the side, place your hands (one on top of the other) on the left side of the rib cage where it is the widest and within 2 to 3 inches of the point of the elbow. Depress the rib cage 1.5 to 2 inches at a rate of 80 to 100 times per minute. **Right:** To compress the chest of a medium to large dog lying on his back, place your hands (one on top of the other) on the sternum, which is the bone lying in the middle of the rib cage. Depress the sternum about 1.5 to 2 inches at a rate of 80 to 100 times per minute.

but is very poor and shallow and your pet is still not responsive, continue artificial respiration at a rate of 10 to 15 times per minute and monitor the pulse every minute.

If you find your *dog does not have a pulse and is still not breathing, you must coordinate chest compressions with the artificial respiration.* The chest should be compressed in a ''cough-like manner'' so that the pressure within the chest is increased and decreased rapidly. To perform chest compressions in a small dog, see Figure 1-18 [Bottom]. To perform chest compressions in medium to large dogs, see Figure 1-19. In large deep chested dogs such as Irish Setters and Greyounds, CPR is more effective if the dog is lying on its back and compressions are done on the sternum, although it may be hard to keep your dog in this position (see Figure 1-19 [Right]).

If you are by yourself performing CPR and you have a small dog, try to coordinate chest compressions and artificial respiration so that breaths can be given *during* the compressions at a rate of at least 20 times per minute. With a compression rate of 120 times per minute, a breath given with every sixth compression would produce the proper respiration rate. In medium to large dogs, respiration and compressions cannot be performed together; two breaths should be given immediately after 15 compressions at a rate of at least 12 per minute.

If you are performing CPR with a partner:

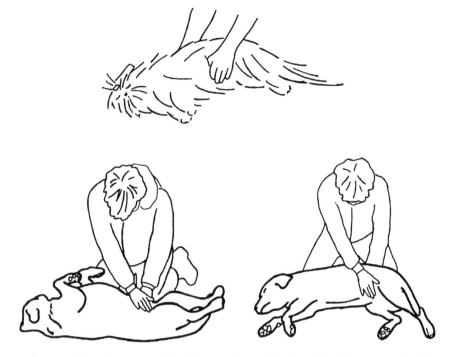

Figure 1-20: Top: To compress the abdomen of a small dog from the side, press gently with the flat of your hand on the left at the level of the umbilicus (midabdomen) about 1 inch. **Bottom left:** To compress the abdomen of a medium to large dog lying on his back, press gently with the flat of your hand on the umbilicus (midabdomen) about 1.5 inches. **Bottom right:** To compress the abdomen of a large dog from the side, press gently with the flat of your hand on the left at the level of the umbilicus (midabdomen) about 1.5 inches.

1. One person will give artificial respiration while the other person does the chest compressions.
2. The chest compressions should be given at the same rate as if you were by yourself (see above).
3. Artificial respiration should be given during chest compressions with every second or third compression, regardless of the size of your dog, thus increasing the oxygen flow to the lungs.

If you have the assistance of two other people:

1. CPR can be given by two people and the third person can give abdominal compressions between each chest compression (see Figure 1-20).
2. The abdominal compression rate will equal the chest compression rate since they are given alternately.
3. The abdomen should be compressed just as the chest compression

is ending so that pressure is maintained on either the chest or abdomen, but never on both at the same time.

4. Abdominal compressions given in this way increase the flow of blood to the brain and heart. You should check for a pulse or a heartbeat every 2 minutes during the resuscitation.

You should continue to give CPR until:

(1) a veterinarian can take over,
(2) you become exhausted and cannot go on, or
(3) you feel a heartbeat or pulse.

If a pulse does return, you must continue artificial respiration as it may take a while before your dog will breathe independently. If your dog does recover before you can get to a veterinarian, remember to continue to monitor the pulse and respiration until your dog can be thoroughly examined by a veterinarian.

Summary

When faced with a **nonresponsive dog,** remember to **check the ABC's** (airway, breathing and circulation) and use the appropriate CPR technique for each situation.

Pulse, no breathing

Small dog	20–25 breaths/minute (1 breath every 3 seconds)
Medium and large dog	15–20 breaths/minute (1 breath every 4 seconds)

No pulse, no breathing

Small dog	120–150 compressions/minute (2 compressions every 1 second)
1 person:	1 breath during every 6th chest compression
2 people:	1 breath during every 3rd chest compression
3 people:	1 breath during every 3rd chest compression (abdominal compression interposed with chest compression)

Medium and large dog	80–100 compressions/minute (15 compressions every 10 seconds)
1 person:	2 breaths after every 15 compressions
2 people:	1 breath during every 3rd chest compression
3 people:	1 breath during every 3rd chest compression (abdominal compression interposed with chest compression)

SECTION 4: DROWNING

Although most dogs are excellent swimmers, drownings may still occur. Usually drowning is the result of a dog jumping into a swimming pool and then being unable to get out; but drowning may also occur when a dog becomes exhausted or panics while swimming in a lake or river.

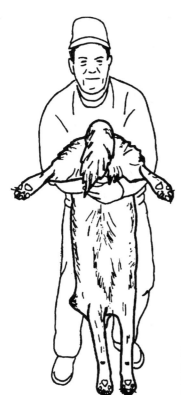

Figure 1-21: To remove water from your dog's lungs, hold him upside down by placing your arms around his lower abdomen and gently sway back and forth for 30 seconds.

The lungs will fill rapidly with water making it impossible for the dog to breathe. When coming to the aid of a drowning dog, your *first step must be to remove as much water as possible from the lungs*.

First Aid

- Open the airway (see Figure 1-15).
- Next hold your dog upside down by placing your arms around the dog's abdomen (see Figure 1-21).
- Lay your dog on his side and check for an open airway again before beginning CPR.
- If your dog does recover from the drowning incident, remember to continue to monitor the pulse and respiration until he can be thoroughly examined by your veterinarian.

SECTION 5: CHOKING

Dogs can be fairly indiscriminate about what they put in their mouths. They may pick up and try to swallow all manner of objects: food, small balls, stones, clothes, toys, etc. Most of the time, your dog will probably be successful at dislodging the object by a forceful cough. But sometimes, the object becomes stuck and leaves your dog in a choking fit, unable to remove it. If the object is not removed quickly, your dog will not be able to breathe well and may become unconscious. From this point, the dog might stop breathing altogether and need to be resuscitated. This section will explain how to take immediate action to prevent this course of events from ever happening.

As with CPR, the first aid method for choking can be done in the car. Being able to perform this technique while on the way to the emergency clinic or veterinary hospital will save you precious moments should your dog become unconscious and need to be resuscitated.

Signs of Choking:

- Forceful coughing
- Eyes bulging
- Pawing at mouth

First Aid

Conscious Dog

- If you are by yourself, hold your dog's mouth open and look inside (see Figure 1-22 [Left]). If you can see the object, try to remove it.
- If you have help, one person should hold your dog's mouth open, while the other person looks inside and removes the object (see Figure 1-22 [Right]).
- If you cannot see the object, lay your dog on his side with lowered head and elevated hindquarters.
- For a small dog, place one hand just below the sternum or rib cage and the other hand along the back (see Figure 1-23 [Top]). Press in and up.
- For a large dog, place both hands just beneath the rib cage and press in and up (see Figure 1-23 [Bottom left]).
- You should continue pressing until your dog either coughs up the object or becomes unconscious.

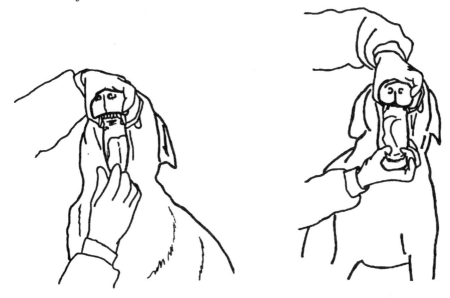

Figure 1-22: Left: To look in your dog's mouth when you are by youself, place one hand on the upper jaw with the thumb on one side and the rest of the fingers on the other side. Use your other hand to open the lower jaw, keeping your thumb and forefinger free to remove foreign objects from the mouth. **Right:** To look in your dog's mouth when you have assistance, one person should place one hand on the upper jaw, with the thumb on one side and the rest of the fingers on the other side. The other hand should open the lower jaw with the thumb on one side and the rest of the fingers on the other side. The second person can then get a good look inside and remove any foreign objects.

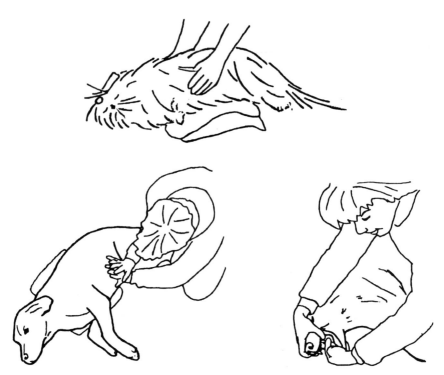

Figure 1-23: Top: For a small dog who is choking, lay your dog on his side with lowered head and elevated hindquarters. Place one hand along the back and the other hand just below the sternum or rib cage, pressing in and up. **Bottom left:** For a large dog who is choking, lay your dog on his side with lowered head and elevated hindquarters. Place both hands just beneath the rib cage and press in and up. **Bottom right:** To check the mouth for foreign objects, place one hand on the upper jaw, with your thumb on one side and the rest of your fingers on the other side. With your other hand, push down on the lower jaw, keeping your index finger free to sweep back into the mouth.

Unconscious Dog
- Lay your dog on his side with lowered head and elevated hindquarters.
- Keep the airway open and tongue pulled out to the side (see Figure 1-15).
- All depending on the size of the dog, perform two compressions in the same manner as if the dog were conscious (see Figure 1-23 [Top or Bottom left]).
- Next check the mouth for foreign bodies with a finger sweep (see Figure 1-23 [Bottom right]).
- Then give two breaths (see Figure 1-17).
- Repeat the cycle of compressions, finger sweep and artificial respirations until your dog is breathing on his own.
- Every few minutes, check for a pulse.

Summary

The two basic first aid techniques for a choking dog depend upon whether the dog is conscious or not. Both methods incorporate a Heimlich-like maneuver to remove the object lodged in the airway. For an unconscious dog, two more steps are added: (1) a finger sweep motion to check for a foreign body and (2) artificial respiration to increase the amount of oxygen taken into the lungs.

SECTION 6: SHOCK AND SEVERE BLEEDING

Shock occurs when the circulatory system fails to deliver blood throughout the body. **It may be caused by severe bleeding, severe burns, electric shock, gastric torsion, prolonged vomiting and diarrhea, allergic reactions (anaphylactic), snake bites, diabetes or any traumatic injury.** Severe blood loss will be discussed in this section; the other causes will be discussed in Chapter 3. *Shock requires immediate attention because, if left untreated, it can rapidly progress to unconsciousness and death.*

Shock

How will you know if your dog is in shock? It may be hard to tell in the very early stages, but as you assess your dog you will note certain problems which, when taken together, mean that shock is beginning:

- Increased respiration rate
- Increased pulse rate
- Gums will appear pale or slightly reddened
- Capillary refill time is more than 2 seconds
- General weakness
- Restless, anxious behavior

As shock progresses, you will see these signs:

- Slow, shallow respiratory rate
- Irregular pulse
- Gum color is very pale to blue
- Capillary refill time is longer than 4 seconds
- Pupils become dilated
- Very weak to unresponsive to unconscious state
- Very cold body temperature (below 98°F)

Obviously, if you see the late stages of shock, your dog is close to death.

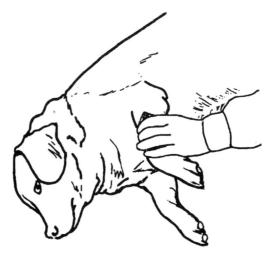

Figure 1-24: To apply direct pressure to a bleeding wound, press down with your bare hand or with a pad held in your hand.

First Aid

- Resuscitate (see CPR, Section 3) and stop severe bleeding.
- Place a blanket or towel under and on top of your dog to prevent loss of body heat.
- Confine your dog.
- Transport your dog immediately to a veterinary clinic (see Section 2 of this chapter).
- Remember that shock can develop or become worse during transport.
- **Do not** give your dog anything to drink.
- **Do not** allow your dog to move around.

Severe Bleeding

Bleeding may be external or internal. If your dog has been hit by a car or has had some other major injury and you see no signs of blood, you shouldn't assume that there is no bleeding. Because there may be internal bleeding, you should have your dog checked by your veterinarian. If you do notice bleeding, especially large amounts of blood over a short period of time, you should follow the techniques listed below in the order

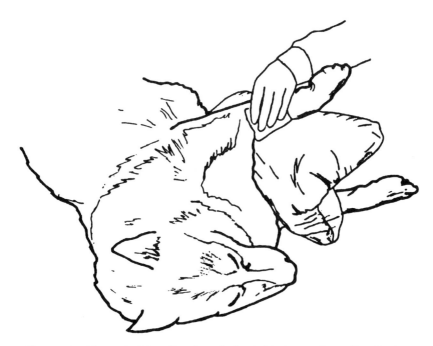

Figure 1-25: Elevate the injured leg above the level of the heart using a pillow, blanket, or towel. This technique can be combined with direct pressure.

given until the bleeding stops. These techniques are more effective when combined and can all be performed in a car.

1) Direct Pressure: To apply direct pressure, see Figure 1-24. It is better to use a dressing than your bare hand as the cloth will allow a clot to form and can be incorporated into the bandage (see Chapter 4, Section 2). *Never remove a pad/cloth which is soaked with blood as you will disturb the clot and bleeding will start anew.* Instead, place a new pad or cloth on top of the soaked one. The bleeding should stop within 1 to 2 minutes.

2) Elevate: Only elevate the injured leg if you suspect that it is not broken (see Figure 1-25).

3) Pressure Points: If the bleeding is not controlled by direct pressure and elevation, you may also use a pressure point to help stop the bleeding. This is a point where pressure is applied to the main artery supplying the bleeding area. In some cases, you may need help to apply direct pressure and use a pressure point simultaneously. You should be aware of five major pressure points:

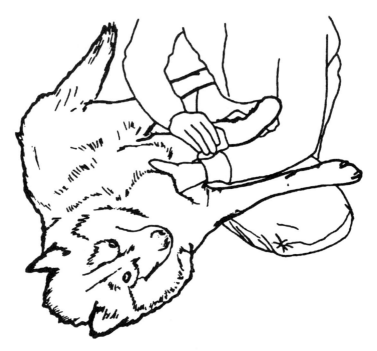

Figure 1-26: To stop severe bleeding on the front leg, place the flat sides of your fingers on the inside of the upper foreleg about halfway between the shoulder and the elbow. Place your thumb on the outside of the foreleg and press your fingers toward the bone. Pressure here is being combined with direct pressure and elevation.

- **Front leg:** For severe bleeding of the front leg, see Figure 1-26.
- **Front foot:** For severe bleeding of the front foot, see Figure 1-27.
- **Back leg:** For severe bleeding of the back leg, see Figure 1-28.
- **Back foot:** For severe bleeding of the back foot, see Figure 1-29.
- **Tail:** For severe bleeding of the tail, see Figure 1-30.

4) Pressure Above and Below the Wound: If bleeding is still not controlled and you have help, then in addition to the above methods, pressure may be applied both above and below the wound (see Figure 1-31).

5) Tourniquet: Tourniquets are very dangerous and may easily cause the loss of a limb. The use of a tourniquet should be reserved for situations where bleeding is very severe, all other methods have been tried *and* the leg is not expected to be saved. To make a tourniquet, see Figure 1-32. The tourniquet should be left on until a veterinarian can take it off.

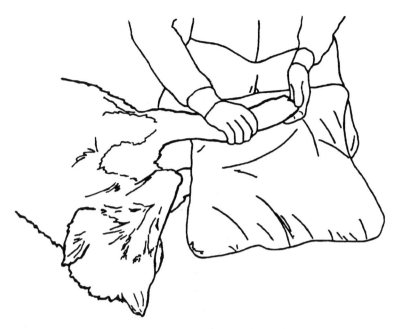

Figure 1-27: To stop severe bleeding on the front paw, place your thumb on the inside of the lower foreleg, just above the paw. Press firmly with your thumb.

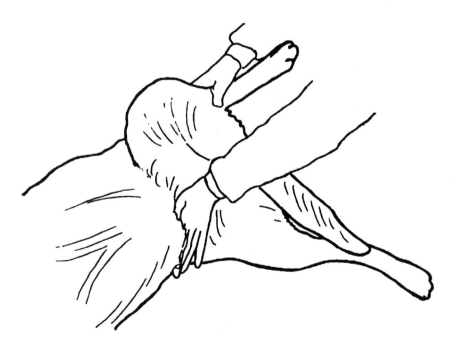

Figure 1-28: To stop severe bleeding on the back leg, press the heel of your hand on the inside of the thigh in the groin area. This is the same place where the pulse is taken.

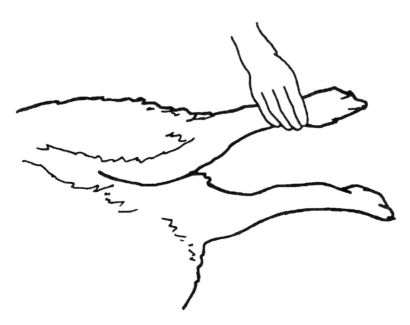

Figure 1-29: To stop severe bleeding on the back paw, place the flat sides of your fingers on the front of the leg, just above the paw. Place your thumb on the back of the leg and press your fingers and thumb together tightly.

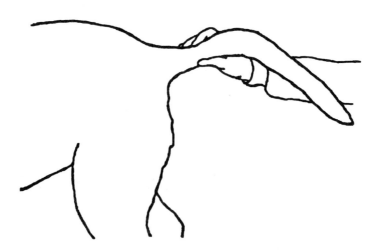

Figure 1-30: To stop severe bleeding on the tail, place your thumb under the middle of the tail and the rest of your fingers around the top of the tail. Press your thumb down tightly.

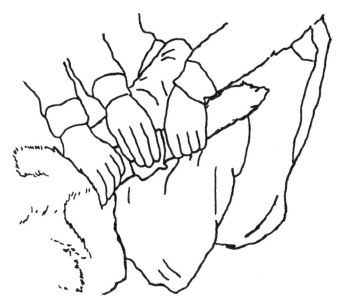

Figure 1-31: To stop severe bleeding which is not controlled by direct pressure, elevation and pressure points, have one person apply direct pressure to the wound itself and pressure below the wound. The other person can then apply pressure above the wound.

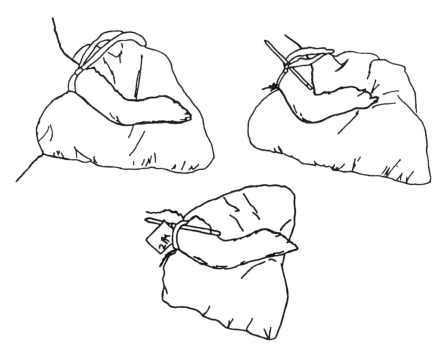

Figure 1-32: Top left: First, place a 6- to 12-inch piece of cloth or gauze around the leg just above the area of severe bleeding and tie a knot. **Top right:** The second step in applying a tourniquet is to tie a pencil or stick into the knot. **Bottom:** The third step is to twist the pencil until the bleeding stops and then to tie the pencil down with another piece of cloth so it stays tight. Insert a note bearing the time the tourniquet was applied.

SUMMARY

In summary, knowing how to approach an emergency can save you time in situations where you need to act without hesitation. Understanding the basic first aid techniques for such life threatening conditions as cardio-pulmonary arrest, shock, drowning and choking will enable you to help your dog immediately and thus greatly increase chances of the dog's survival.

2

What to Do Second:
The Head-to-Toe Exam

ONCE YOU HAVE PERFORMED basic life saving tech-
niques and your dog's condition is stable, take a closer look at your dog
to make sure there are no other problems.

For example, a dog who has been hit by a car may have severe
internal injuries which you can't see, but ones you might be able to detect
on exam. Once you understand how to check your dog and know what
to look for, you can do a head-to-toe exam in 5 to 10 minutes, identify
other problems your dog might have and then give the appropriate first
aid. As with the basic life saving techniques, the physical exam can be
performed in a car on the way to the emergency clinic or veterinary
hospital.

In this chapter, we will learn how to examine the major body systems
quickly. The common emergencies for each system will be described and
first aid measures will be detailed. In all cases, be sure to contact your
veterinarian if you have access to a telephone to determine if your dog
should be seen immediately.

Many of the first aid methods in the sections to follow involve
bandages. The reader will be referred to the bandaging section (Chapter
4, Section 2) in these instances. Many bandages, especially those applied
to the head or the extremities, may stay on much better if your dog wears
an Elizabethan collar. These collar are discussed in the bandaging section.

Before you begin the head-to-toe exam, take the temperature, pulse and respiratory rate (see Triage, Chapter 1, Section 1) if you have not already done so.

SECTION 1: EYES

Exam

To start the exam, ask yourself if your dog can see. A sighted dog can walk around without bumping into things. If there is any question in your mind, change the positions of some chairs to see if your dog can still maneuver without bumping.

Next, look at the eyes. If only one eye is injured, compare the injured eye to the normal eye. Check the following parameters:

1. Pupil size (see Figure 2-1)
2. Response to light
3. Eyeball position
4. Excessive blinking or tearing

To check the pupil size, shine a flashlight into your dog's eye (checking one eye at a time). The pupil should become smaller (*constrict*). When you remove the light, the pupil should return to the original size. If you bring your dog into a dimly lit room, the pupil should become larger (*dilate*). When you shine the flashlight into your dog's eye, you should also note her behavioral response to the light. If she turns away or starts blinking or tearing, her eye may be painful. You can check the position of the eyeball from the front and the side. The eyeball should be neither sunken in nor pushed out. Your dog's eyes should be clear with no noticeable discharge. If you do see a discharge, note the color and consistency (for example, yellow and thick).

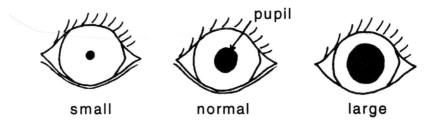

pupil

small   normal   large

Figure 2-1: Pupil size in room light.

Emergencies

Glaucoma

Glaucoma occurs when the pressure within the eye increases. The signs of this disease are:

- Dilated pupil
- Enlarged eyeball
- Pupil which slowly constricts or does not constrict at all
- Afraid to look into the light
- Tearing
- Steamy appearance to the eye

Although there is no first aid as such, it is important to be able to recognize the signs of this disease and have your dog examined immediately, as permanent damage to the eye can occur within a few days.

Prolapse of the eye

The eyeball is prolapsed when it is partially or fully out of the socket. It usually occurs in conjunction with a fight, fall or being hit by a car.

First Aid

- Cover the eye with a sterile pad or cloth which has been moistened in cold sterile saline or cold water.
- Bandage the eye to the socket area by loosely wrapping with gauze and adhesive (see Chapter 4 and Figure 4-6).
- Do not attempt to push the eye back into the socket.

Foreign object in the eye

A stone, piece of glass, BB pellet, sand or similar small object may become lodged in your dog's eye. Look carefully to see if the object has penetrated the eye. The signs of this condition are:

- Presence of a foreign object in the eye
- Blinking
- Squinting
- Tearing
- Turning away from the light

- Lift the upper eyelid and look very carefully for the foreign object (see Figure 2-2 [Top left]).
- If the eye is clear, relax the skin of the upper eyelid and pull down gently on the skin of the lower eyelid using the thumb of the other hand. Again, look carefully for the object.

For a nonpenetrating object:
- Wash it out by gently pouring sterile saline or cool water onto the eye surface for a few minutes (see Figure 2-2 [Top right]).
- Another method is to ease the foreign object carefully out of the eye by using a cotton swab moistened with cool, fresh water (see Figure 2-2 [Bottom]).
- If you cannot remove the object from the eye, place a sterile pad or cloth over the eye and bandage as shown in Figures 4-6 in Chapter 4, Section 2. The bandage will prevent further trauma until the object is removed by your veterinarian.

For a penetrating object:
- Do not attempt to remove the object.
- To prevent further trauma, put an Elizabethan collar on your dog (see Figure 4-15 in Chapter 4, Section 2) until she can be examined by your veterinarian.

Trauma to the eye surface

The surface of the eye (cornea) may become irritated by scratches from cats, chemicals which burn or the presence of foreign objects in the eye (see discussion above). You might suspect the cornea has been irritated if the eye appears normal except for the following signs:

- Blinking
- Squinting
- Redness
- Tearing
- Turning away from the light

First Aid

Scratches:
- Cover the eye with a sterile pad or clean cloth.

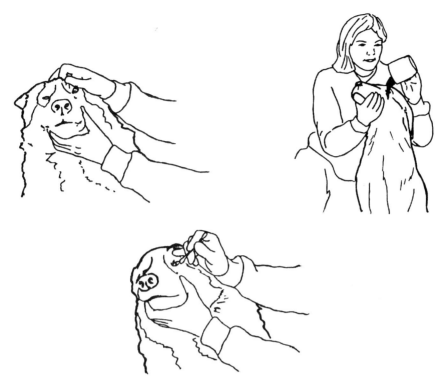

Figure 2-2: Top left: To look for an object in the eye, place one hand directly above the eye while the other hand holds the lower jaw. With the hand above the eye, pull gently up on the skin. To check the lower surface of the eye, relax the skin above the eye and use the thumb of the hand on the lower jaw to pull down the skin just below the eye. **Top right:** To wash a foreign object out of the eye, gently pour cool water or sterile saline onto the eye surface for a few minutes. **Bottom:** To remove a foreign object from the eye with a cotton swab, first moisten the swab with cool water or sterile saline. Holding the swab in one hand, carefully ease the foreign object out of the eye using the tip of the swab while the other hand holds the lower muzzle for restraint.

- Bandage loosely to the head, leaving the normal eye unbandaged (see Figure 4-6 in Chapter 4, Section 2).

Chemical Burns:
- The chemical should be washed out immediately.
- Pour plenty of cool water onto the eye surface for at least 5 minutes (see Figure 2-2 [Top right]).
- Cover the injured eye with a sterile pad or clean cloth and bandage loosely to the head, leaving the normal eye free (see Figure 4-6 in Chapter 4, Section 2).

Trauma to the lids

The eyelids may become traumatized during any severe injury, for example being hit by a car or being involved in a fight with another animal. The lids will appear:

- Torn
- Bruised
- Swollen

First Aid

- Hold a cold compress (not ice) over the lid for 5 to 10 minutes to reduce swelling.
- Cover with a clean, dry pad and bandage loosely to the head, leaving the unaffected eye unbandaged (see Figure 4-6 in Chapter 4, Section 2).

Blood in the eye

Severe head trauma or penetrating eye wounds may cause blood in the eye. It may clear on its own in 7 to 14 days without any further problems or it may be complicated by glaucoma or retinal detachment.

First Aid

- Since movement may increase the bleeding, keep your dog as quiet and confined as possible until she can be examined.

SECTION 2: EARS

Exam

To check the ears, first determine if your dog can hear. Stand behind your dog, clap your hands loudly and look for a response. Next check the color of the inside of the ear. It should be pink. Be sure to examine both the outside and inside of the ear for the following: bite wounds, swellings, plant materials and ticks.

Emergencies

Hematoma

A hematoma is a swelling which contains blood. They are usually caused by violent head shaking or develop from bite wounds and may be on the inside or outside of the ear. The major sign is a soft, fluctuant swelling on the ear.

First Aid

- If your dog cannot be examined by your veterinarian immediately, bandage the affected ear to the head (see Figure 4-7 in Chapter 4, Section 2) to prevent the hematoma from enlarging.

Foreign objects

Foreign objects such as plant material and ticks may become embedded in the ear canal. Depending upon how far into the ear canal the foreign object has gone, your dog may have some or all of the following signs:

- Head shaking
- Rotating the head with the affected ear down
- Falling and circling to the affected side
- Inability to eat and drink normally
- Fever

First Aid

- If the foreign object is visible and your dog will stay still, remove it with tweezers or your fingers and save it for identification (see Figure 2-3).
- If you suspect a foreign object in the ear and have a dog with pendulous ears, bandage the ear to the head (see Figure 4-7 in Chapter 4, Section 2) until your dog can be examined. This will prevent further injury to the ear, including hematoma formation.

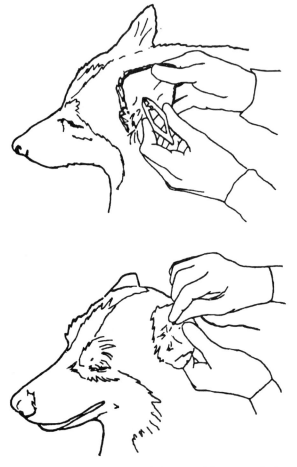

Figure 2-3: A foreign object may be removed from your dog's ear via either tweezers **(Top)** or your fingers **(Bottom)**. To remove a foreign object with a tweezers, grasp the object with the tweezers about the part which is closest to the skin and pull out evenly. To remove a foreign object with your fingers, cradle the object with your thumb and first two fingers and pull out evenly.

Lacerations

Your dog's ear may become lacerated or torn from fighting with another animal. The major sign will be a very bloody ear.

First Aid

- Stop the bleeding by direct pressure (see Chapter 1, Section 6).
- Leave the cloth on the clot and bandage the ear (see Figures 4-7 and 4-8 in Chapter 4, Section 2).

SECTION 3: NOSE

Exam

To examine the nose and nasal passageways, observe the breathing and shine a flashlight into the nostrils. Normal breathing is in and out through the nose at 10 to 30 breaths per minute. Your dog should not be panting unless the environment is hot or stressful. When you shine a flashlight into the nostrils, they should be clear and free of discharge. If discharge is present, note the type (blood, pus, water) and if it is coming from one or both nostrils. The nose itself may or may not be moist.

Emergencies

Nosebleed

Blood coming from one or both nostrils is usually caused by a traumatic injury.

First Aid

- Keep your dog quiet and confined.
- Apply cold compresses to the nose. Do not use ice as it may cause freezing.
- Do not tilt your dog's head back to lessen the bleeding, as the dog may choke on the blood.
- Do not pack the nostrils with gauze, as this may cause sneezing and more bleeding.

Foreign objects

These usually consist of plant material which has lodged in the nasal passageways. The signs you may see are:

- Frequent episodes of sneezing or snorting
- Banging of the head

First Aid

- If you can see a foreign object, try to remove it with tweezers (see Figure 2-4).
- If you cannot remove the foreign object or don't see one, have your dog examined by your veterinarian.

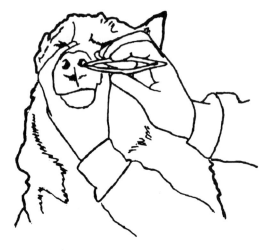

Figure 2-4: To remove a foreign object from the nose, steady the muzzle with one hand and use the tweezers with your other hand.

SECTION 4: MOUTH/THROAT

Exam

To examine the mouth and throat, check the gums, the teeth, the tongue and chewing and swallowing. The gum color should be pale pink and the capillary refill time should be less than 2 seconds (see Chapter 1, Section 1). Use a flashlight to take a good look in the mouth. Watch your dog eat and drink. The dog should not drool (excessive saliva) and should be chewing and swallowing food normally. You might suspect your dog has a painful mouth if she appears hungry and avoids food and water. Under the same circumstances, your dog might extend her neck or choke while trying to swallow.

Emergencies

Foreign objects

Some dogs, especially puppies, may indiscriminately try to eat fish-hooks, stones, string, balls, bones, needles or whatever looks good at that particular moment. Depending upon how far down in the throat the foreign object gets, you may see signs of:

- Drooling
- Blood from the mouth
- Neck extension on swallowing
- Choking on swallowing

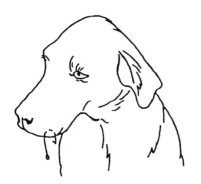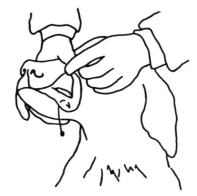

Figure 2-5: Left: To remove a fishhook with the barbed hook end exposed, cut the hook end off with a wire cutter and then carefully remove the straight edge of the hook. If there is any resistance, stop pulling and let your veterinarian remove it. **Right:** In dealing with a fishhook with the barbed end embedded, do not pull it or attempt to push it through the skin. This must be removed by your veterinarian.

- Appetite but not eating or drinking
- Vomiting

First Aid for Fishhooks

- If the barbed hook end is exposed, see Figure 2-5 [Left].
- If the barbed hook end is embedded, see Figure 2-5 [Right].

First Aid for String or Tinsel

- First check to see if any part of the string or tinsel has been swallowed.
- If part has been swallowed, do not pull the remaining piece, as you may cause severe damage. It must be surgically removed by your veterinarian.
- If the string or tinsel is loose in the mouth, remove it slowly and carefully. If you feel resistance, stop pulling and have your dog examined by your veterinarian.

First Aid for Other Foreign Objects

- If you can see the foreign object, remove it carefully with your hand, needlenose pliers or tweezers (see Figure 1-22 [Left]).

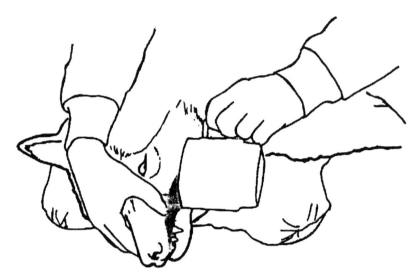

Figure 2-6: With one hand, lift up your dog's lip toward the back of his mouth. The other hand holds a cup or a slowly running hose.

- If the foreign object is not right at the front of the mouth, have a friend hold your dog's mouth open while you remove the foreign object (see Figure 1-22 [Right]).

Mouth burns

The mouth of your dog may become burned by chewing on an electric cord or by contact with a caustic chemical. Chewing on an electric cord can cause electric shock and will be discussed in Chapter 3, Section 8. Signs of mouth burns due to chemicals are:

- Drooling
- Avoidance of food and water
- Avoidance of petting around the mouth and face

First Aid

- Lay your dog on his side, with neck resting on a pillow so his nose is down.
- Lift up the lip to expose the teeth (see Figure 2-6).
- Flush large amounts of cool water through the mouth by using a cup or a slow-running hose.

52

Blood from the mouth

This emergency is usually due to a severe trauma of some sort, usually an auto accident or a fight. The blood may be coming from a wound in the mouth (such as a broken tooth) or may be due to internal bleeding or a severe head injury.

First Aid

- Use a flashlight and try to find where the blood is coming from. Check the teeth.
- If you can see the wound in the mouth, apply a cold compress with pressure until the bleeding stops.
- If you do not see a source of the blood, notify your veterinarian because your dog should be examined immediately.
- Look for signs of shock (Chapter 1, Section 6). Monitor gum color, refill time and pulse.
- Do not tilt the head back to stop the bleeding, as your dog may choke on the blood.

Tracheal collapse

The trachea is a tube-like part of the respiratory system which allows air to move from the mouth or nose into the lungs. If the tube is too small or if the supporting tissues are too soft, the airway may not be able to remain open. Tracheal collapse occurs most often in the Toy breeds of dogs such as the Yorkshire Terrier, Pomeranian, Chihuahua, and Toy and Miniature Poodle. It can be brought on by excitement, exercise, manual pressure on the trachea and drinking and eating. The following signs, when taken together, may mean that your dog has a **collapsed trachea:**

- Cough which sounds like a goose honk
- Mouth breathing
- Extended head and neck

First Aid

- Calm and confine your dog.

NOTE: **Make an appointment with your veterinarian for a thorough examination of your dog. Keep a record of the coughing spells and the circumstances causing them.**

SECTION 5: CHEST

Exam

1. To examine the chest, check the following: chest wall symmetry, breathing, pain or wounds on the chest.
2. To look at the symmetry of the chest wall, stand behind your dog. As she breathes, you should see both sides of the chest rise and fall equally.
3. Listen closely to the breathing. The rate varies between 10 and 30 breaths per minute (see Chapter 1, Section 1).
4. Is your dog having difficulty breathing at rest or during exercise? Difficult breathing is heavy, may be noisy and may be at a faster rate than normal.
5. To check for pain, press gently on the ribs with your fingers. If your dog is in pain, she may yelp, snap or try to move away.
6. Finally, use your fingertips to feel along the fur over the chest for dried blood or puncture wounds.

Emergencies

Rib fractures

The ribs may become fractured in any case of chest trauma. You will see the following signs:

- Unsymmetrical chest wall. *The side which doesn't rise as much may have a fractured rib.*
- Painful breathing.
- Pain when the rib is pressed.
- May or may not be a wound.

First Aid

- Keep your dog quiet and confined.
- Lay your dog on her side with the fractured rib down. In this way, the fractured rib will exert no pressure on the lung which will be ventilated the most (the top one).

Chest wounds

Chest wounds occur with any severe trauma to the chest wall. The wounds may create an opening all the way to the chest cavity (open) or stay outside the chest cavity (closed).

The signs of an open chest wound are the following:

- Difficulty breathing.
- Blood, muscles of the chest wall are exposed.
- Air being sucked in and out of the chest cavity (it may be difficult to hear this).
- May have fractured ribs.

First Aid

- Do not wash or clean.
- Soak a pad or cloth in sterile saline or cool water and place the pad over the wound immediately after your dog breathes out.
- Bandage firmly (see Figure 4-10 in Chapter 4, Section 2).
- Make sure your dog can breathe normally with the bandage in place.
- Maintain an open airway if necessary.
- Monitor breathing until your dog can be examined.

CLOSED WOUNDS
The signs of a closed chest wound are the following:

- May or may not have a break in the skin.
- Difficulty breathing.
- Will not hear air being sucked in.
- May have fractured ribs.

First Aid

- If there is a break in the skin, treat as for an open chest wound, since there may be an opening all the way to the chest cavity.
- If there is not a break in the skin, keep your dog confined and quiet and monitor breathing until she can be examined.

SECTION 6: ABDOMEN

Exam

To check the abdominal area of your dog, look at the symmetry of the abdomen as well as feeling for pain and wounds.

1. Stand behind your dog and look at both sides of the abdomen; they should be about the same size.
2. Press your hands gently down on the abdomen. A dog with a painful abdomen will hold her belly in a tight, tense fashion and will stand with her back slightly arched up. Alternatively, she may want to lie down on a cool surface.
3. If your dog has severe pain in the upper abdomen, she may lower her front end while keeping her back end raised.
4. To check for dried blood and wounds, place your fingertips on the middle of your dog's belly.
5. Move them slowly over the skin and fur until you have covered the entire abdomen.

Emergencies

Bloat (Gastric Torsion)

This emergency will be discussed in Chapter 3, Section 4.

Gastric foreign objects

Some objects which dogs may put in their mouths will actually make it all the way down to their stomachs, such as stones, buttons, pins and, in one case, a small kitchen knife! They may cause obstructions or puncture internal organs if not removed. You may see the following signs if your dog has swallowed a foreign object:

- Tightened abdominal muscles
- Vomiting
- Rapid pulse
- Loss of appetite
- Fever
- Abdominal distension (with an obstruction only)
- Reduced production of feces (with an obstruction only)

Nonpenetrating injuries

These are injuries to the abdomen where the skin is not broken. They are caused mostly by automobile accidents and include the rupture or bruising of abdominal organs. Generally, the signs seen are the same as with gastric foreign bodies (without an obstruction) but will vary depending upon which organ is ruptured or bruised:

- Bloody urine or no urine (bladder or kidney damage)
- Pain over the part of the abdomen closest to the head (spleen or liver damage)

There is no first aid as such for gastric foreign objects or nonpenetrating injuries. However, if you suspect either of these conditions, you should have your dog examined immediately by your veterinarian.

Penetrating injuries

Arrows, knives and gunshot are the common causes of penetrating injuries of the abdomen. The signs you may see are:

- Rapid pulse
- Rapid breathing
- Severe abdominal pain
- Protruding abdominal organs
- Shock

First Aid

- Treat shock (see Chapter 1, Section 6) on the way to your veterinarian.
- If there are protruding abdominal organs, place a clean cloth which has been wet with sterile saline or cool water around the protruding organs and wrap these against the abdomen. Do not try to push the protruding organs back into the abdomen and do not wash the wound.
- If a knife is penetrating the abdomen, it can be pulled out. Once you have pulled the knife out, apply a pad over the wound and bandage (see Figure 4-10 in Chapter 4, Section 2). Do not wash first.
- Do not remove any sharp objects which may cause more damage upon removal (for example, arrows). Simply bandage around this area without washing as you would for a knife wound.

Sudden stomach upset (gastritis)

Your dog may get gastritis when she eats garbage, spoiled food or table scraps. The signs include:

- Vomiting
- Diarrhea (sometimes with blood)

- Dehydration
- Pain in the upper abdomen

First Aid

- If your dog appears dehydrated (see Figure 1-4 and 1-5 [Left]) have her seen by your veterinarian immediately.
- If your dog is not dehydrated and is vomiting, withhold food and water for 12-24 hours and then offer small amounts.
- If your dog is not dehydrated and has diarrhea but no vomiting, withhold food for 12-24 hours and restrict water to small amounts offered often. At the end of the 12-24 hours, offer small amounts of food along with the water.
- If the vomiting/diarrhea persists during the 12-24 hours or begins again upon feeding, have your dog examined by your veterinarian.

NOTE: **For more information on vomiting/diarrhea, see Chapter 3, Section 13.**

Rectal Prolapse

The rectum may prolapse in dogs who strain due to constipation, tumors or giving birth. It may also occur in young puppies. The signs seen are:

- Round mass of tissue protruding from the anus
- Color of the tissue is initially red, turning dark red later

First Aid

- Wrap a clean cloth which has been moistened with cool water around the cylindrical mass. This will keep the tissue moist until it can be manipulated to its normal position by your veterinarian.

SECTION 7: EXTREMITIES

Exam

Due to trauma, mostly from automobile accidents, both the front and hind legs of your dog may be badly injured.

To examine the legs:

1. Watch your dog walk
2. Look at the joints
3. Check for the presence of pain, wounds or broken bones.

As you watch your dog walk, look to see if she favors one leg over the others. Her joints should not be swollen or puffy. To check for pain, press with your fingertips, all along the leg. Lightly pinch the dog's toes to see if she pulls the leg away. This means that the dog can feel the pain. Finally, use a comb or your fingertips to run through the coat looking for dried blood, torn skin or other evidence of wounds.

Emergencies

Fractures

The bones in the legs may break when trauma is severe, such as from auto accidents or falls from high places. If your dog is favoring one leg, she may have a fracture. For a more complete discussion on the topic of fractures, please see Chapter 4, Section 3.

First Aid

- If you suspect a fracture, splint the leg before moving your dog (see Chapter 4, Section 3).

Wounds

The skin, muscles, nerves and blood vessels may become torn or punctured due to bites or a severe trauma, such as auto accidents. Wounds may accompany fractures. For a more complete discussion on the topic of wounds, see Chapter 4, Section 1.

First Aid

- For wounds which are bleeding heavily, first stop the bleeding (see Chapter 1, Section 6) and then bandage (see Chapter 4, Section 2).
- For superficial wounds, clean the wound and then apply a bandage (see Chapter 4, Sections 1 and 2).

NOTE: **If your dog has been in an auto accident or fallen from a high place, check her over thoroughly as she may have suffered severe trauma to other parts of her body.**

SECTION 8: RESPONSIVENESS

Exam

If your dog is behaving differently than she usually does, this may be a clue that something is wrong, even if you found no problems during the rest of the head-to-toe exam.

Make a quick note of your dog's responsiveness. You should check to see if she is alert, depressed, drowsy, hyperexcited or disoriented. If you do see a sudden behavior change, this may be a prelude to severe changes in the nervous system, as seen with seizures or coma. Have your dog examined by your veterinarian to determine a cause. Both seizures and coma are discussed in Chapter 3.

Emergencies

Fainting

Fainting is a sudden loss of consciousness which occurs when the brain does not receive enough oxygen or sugar. Fainting may be caused by heart problems, low blood sugar, hyperventilation (overbreathing) or coughing fits. The major signs are:

- Weakness
- Incoordination
- Loss of consciousness
- Recovery within minutes

Since recovery is usually very rapid, there is no first aid as such. Keep a record of the fainting episodes and include how long they last and under what circumstances the fainting takes place, for example exercising or eating.

SUMMARY

In summary, the head-to-toe exam is a crucial component of the first aid scheme. Performed only when your dog is stabilized, it can alert you to problems which may become serious in a short time. Table 1 contains a list of the parameters to check in each system.

TABLE 2-1 Head-to-Toe Exam

Body Part	Parameters
Eyes	sight pupil size response to light eyeball position excessive blinking or tearing
Ears	hearing bite wounds swellings plant materials ticks
Mouth, Throat	gums teeth tongue chewing swallowing
Chest	chest wall symmetry breathing pain wounds
Abdomen	abdominal symmetry pain wounds
Legs	walking joints pain wounds
Responsiveness	alert depressed drowsy hyperexcited disoriented change in behavior

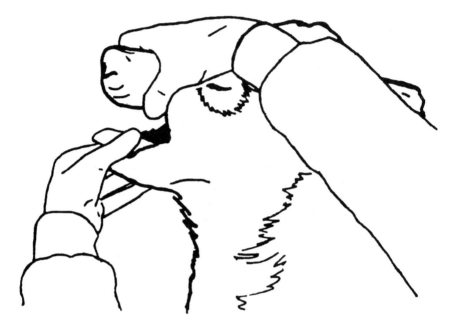

Figure 3-1: In cases where your dog is having breathing difficulties, the airway must be opened. First, extend the head and neck. Open the dog's mouth, pull the tongue forward and clear the mouth of all food, vomit, *etc*.

3

Typical Emergencies
and How to
Handle Them

T HE EMERGENCIES discussed in this chapter all have one common characteristic: if left untreated, they have the potential to cause life threatening problems quickly.

Because they can cause such serious problems, recognizing the signs of these conditions and acting quickly is very important. If you have access to a phone during the emergency, call your veterinarian for advice. This is an important part of first aid for all of the emergencies listed in this chapter. Your veterinarian can tell you if you should bring your dog into the clinic right away or if you can continue to provide care at home.

SECTION 1: ALLERGIC REACTIONS

Allergic Reactions

Two types of allergic reactions which require emergency care are **anaphylactic shock** and **hives.** Both are immediate hypersensitivity reactions, one taking place within a few minutes (anaphylactic shock) and the other taking about twenty minutes to develop (hives).

Anaphylactic Shock

Anaphylactic shock may be caused by a number of different agents, namely drugs, especially antibiotics and local anesthetics, hormones, vaccines, insect bites and food. In a sensitive dog, these substances produce a reaction within minutes which may cause the heart and lungs to collapse. The signs are:

- Difficulty breathing
- Vomiting
- Diarrhea
- Shock
- Coma

First Aid

- Open the airway (see Figure 3-1).
- Perform CPR, if necessary (see Chapter 1, Section 3).
- Treat for shock on the way to your veterinarian (see Chapter 1, Section 6).

Hives

Hives are usually caused by allergies to foods, especially those which are protein-rich such as cow's milk, meat or eggs. In addition, blood transfusions and insect bites may also cause hives in a hypersensitive dog. The signs are localized to the head:

- Redness, swelling in the eyes and mouth
- Intense itching of the swollen areas
- Rubbing face on the ground
- Scratching face with paws
- Difficulty breathing

First Aid

- If the reaction is severe and your dog is having difficulty breathing, notify your veterinarian at once and monitor breathing.
- Put an Elizabethan collar on your dog if he has inflicted rubbing and scratching wounds to his head (see Chapter 4, Section 2).
- Treat the wounds on the face (for general treatment of wounds,

see Chapter 4, Section 1). If you suspect a food allergy, ask your veterinarian for advice on hypoallergenic diets.

SECTION 2: BIRTHING PROBLEMS

Birthing difficulties are usually caused by a small birth canal, weak uterine contractions or an abnormal fetus. Once the puppies are born, they may have difficulty breathing if the mother doesn't lick open the membrane sac. If you can recognize the signs which these problems cause, you can increase the chances that your dog will recover quickly and the puppies will be healthy. The signs of birthing problems are:

- Gestation (the length of the pregnancy) lasting longer than 70 days.
- Failure to whelp 24 hours after the rectal temperature has dropped to lower than 100°F.
- Sixty minutes of strong abdominal contractions *without* the birth of a puppy.
- More than 2 hours between the birth of subsequent puppies.
- Pain or any sign of illness.
- Black, yellow or bloody vaginal discharge is present. (*NOTE:* A greenish-black discharge indicates placental separation, and a puppy should be born within one to two hours.)
- Puppies not breathing immediately after birth.

First Aid

For the mother:
- If you see any signs of birthing problems or if your dog has had any previous birthing problems, call your veterinarian.

For the puppies:
- Open the membrane sac if the mother hasn't done so.
- If the puppy does not start breathing immediately, follow the procedures below in the order given:
  a. use a moistened cotton swab to remove mucus from the mouth and nostrils.
  b. cup the puppy in your hands with the head downward and gently swing to remove more mucus from the nasal passages.
  c. vigorously rub the puppy all over for a minute.
  d. start CPR.

SECTION 3: BITES AND STINGS

This section will cover bites, stings and poisonings from many different types of animals: cats, dogs, wild animals such as raccoons, snakes, ticks, flying insects, spiders, scorpions and lizards.

Domestic/Wild Animal Bites

Bites by domestic or wild animals will cause the following signs:

- Skin is punctured or torn by teeth.
- Area is red and swollen.
- Bleeding will be slight or extensive.

If a dog is not vaccinated for rabies and is bitten by a rabid animal, the dog may also show signs of:

- Sudden change in behavior
- Restlessness
- Viciousness
- Convulsions
- Drooling
- Paralysis

First Aid

- Control bleeding (see Figure 3-2 [Top] and Chapter 1, Section 6).
- Wash wound with soap and water (see Figure 3-2 [Bottom left] and Chapter 4, Section 2).
- Apply a loose bandage (see Figure 3-2 [Bottom right] and Chapter 4, Section 2).
- If your dog shows any signs of rabies or has been exposed to rabies, even if he has been vaccinated, you should notify your local health authority immediately.

Snake Bite

Of all the animals which can cause poisonings in dogs, snakes are responsible for the highest number of cases each year.

Both poisonous and nonpoisonous snakes are widely distributed over the United States. The poisonous snakes which cause a large proportion

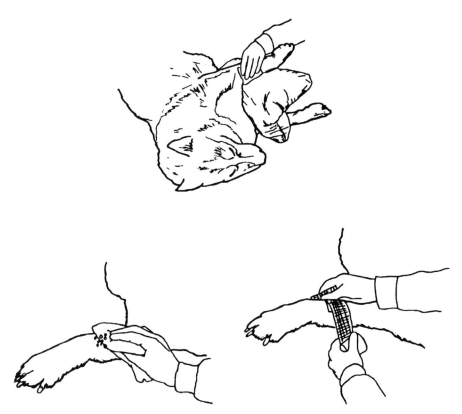

Figure 3-2: Top: Elevate the injured leg above the level of the heart using a pillow, blanket or towel. This technique can be combined with direct pressure. **Bottom left:** To clean a bite wound, use a clean, soft cloth with soap and water. Wash from the center and move outward. Then rinse with water. Wear gloves if your dog was exposed to rabies. **Bottom right:** Cover the bite wound with a pad which has antibiotic ointment on it, followed by gauze. Secure the gauze with adhesive tape (see Chapter 4, Section 2).

of snake bites in dogs are the pit vipers (copperheads, *Agkistrodon contortrix;* rattlesnakes, various species of *Crotalus* and *Sistrurus*; and cottonmouths, *Agkistrodon piscivorus*) and to a lesser extent the coral snakes (*Micruroides euryxanthus* and *Micrurus fulvius*). Table 3-1 lists the distribution of these snakes across the continental United States.

In general, bites from nonpoisonous snakes will look like scratches and won't cause much swelling, redness or pain. The signs of a poisonous snake bite will largely depend on the location of the bite, how much venom is injected and the general health and age of your dog. Most bites occur on the face and legs because dogs are usually sniffing and walking when they encounter a snake. Sick, very young and old dogs may have a longer recovery time. Anaphylactic shock (see Chapter 3, Section 1) may occur in dogs who are sensitive to the venom, but this is rare.

TABLE 3-1 Distribution of Poisonous Snakes in the Continental United States

Copperheads	Alabama Arkansas Connecticut Delaware Florida Georgia Illinois Indiana Kansas	Kentucky Louisiana Maryland Massachusetts Mississippi Missouri New Jersey New York North Carolina	Ohio Oklahoma Pennsylvania South Carolina Tennessee Texas Virginia West Virginia
Coral Snakes	Alabama Arizona Arkansas Florida	Georgia Louisiana Mississippi New Mexico	North Carolina South Carolina Texas
Cottonmouths	Alabama Arkansas Florida Georgia Illinois	Kentucky Louisiana Mississippi Missouri North Carolina	Oklahoma South Carolina Tennessee Texas Virginia
Rattlesnakes	All states *except* Maine		

The signs of a poisonous snake bite are:

- Swelling, pain, redness within 20 minutes at the site of the bite
- Two fang marks (this may be difficult to see due to swelling)
- Difficulty breathing, if bite is on the face or throat
- Lameness, if the bite is on the leg
- Vomiting
- Diarrhea
- Increased pulse
- Shock

First Aid

- Keep your dog as still as possible, as any movement will increase the absorption of the venom. If possible, carry him instead of letting him walk.
- If you have access to a car, transport your dog immediately to the nearest veterinary facility. If you saw the snake, be able to describe it as this will help in the choice of the antivenom. In particular, note the color and pattern of any markings on the snake, and the

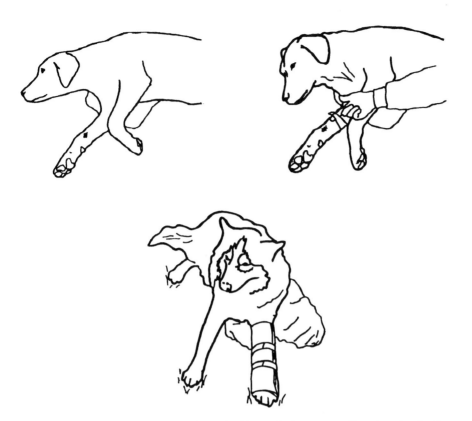

Figure 3-3: Top left; In the case of a snake bite on the leg, use a pillow placed under the dog's upper body to keep the affected leg below the level of the heart. **Top right:** For a snake bite on the leg, tie a piece of cloth or gauze around the leg between the bite and the heart. The cloth should be snug but should allow one finger to fit under it. **Bottom:** To immobilize a leg which has a snake bite on it, wrap newspaper or a magazine around the entire leg and tape closed.

presence or absence of a rattle. **Do not** approach or attempt to kill the snake.

- If your dog is having breathing difficulties, keep the airway open (see Figure 3-1).
- If a leg is bitten, keep it below the level of the heart (see Figure 3-3 [Top left]) and apply pressure using your hand or a flat constricting band (not a tourniquet) between the bite and the heart (see Figure 3-3 [Top right]). You can leave it on for as long as two hours. (Darkening of the skin below the band is an indication that the band is on too tightly.) Then, immobilize the leg with a splint (see Figure 3-3 [Bottom]).
- Treat shock (see Chapter 1, Section 6).

- **Do not** wash the wound, as this may increase the absorption of the venom.
- **Do not** apply ice to the wound, as this may cause the skin to freeze and does not affect the spread of the venom.
- **Do not** make cuts over the wound and attempt to suck the venom out, as you may absorb some of the venom yourself.

NOTE: **If you think your dog was bitten by a nonpoisonous snake and you have access to a car, you should still transport the dog to a veterinary clinic immediately as he will have to be treated for any bacterial infections which may develop.**

Ticks

If your dog has ever been outside, especially near or in wooded areas, then he has been exposed to ticks. Ticks may be found anywhere on your dog but usually are attached to the head, neck and between the toes. In this section, I will discuss three important tick diseases which affect dogs: Tick Paralysis, Lyme Disease and Rocky Mountain Spotted Fever. Since the first aid procedures are generally the same for all three diseases, they will be discussed together.

Tick Paralysis

The ticks which produce this disease are the eastern wood or American dog tick (*Dermancentor variabilis*) and the western mountain or Rocky Mountain wood tick (*Dermancentor andersoni*). Once they are attached, these ticks will inject a toxin through their saliva which will cause the following signs:

Early
- Generalized weakness
- Fever
- Incoordination

Late
- Paralysis
- Difficulty breathing

Lyme Disease

This disease occurs when a tick of the genus *Ixodes* transmits a bacterium, *Borrelia burgdorferi*, through its saliva while attached to a dog.

The ticks which can transmit this disease are distributed in the Northeast (deer tick, *Ixodes dammini*), in the West and Midwest (California black-eyed tick, *Ixodes pacificus*) and in the South (black-legged tick, *Ixodes scapularis*). The tick must be attached to the dog for at least 2 days before infection takes place. Once infection takes place, the following signs are seen:

- Weakness
- Sudden lameness
- Swollen and painful joints
- Fever
- Depression
- Reluctance to move

Rocky Mountain Spotted Fever

The ticks which produce this disease are the same as those which cause tick paralysis: the eastern wood or American dog tick (*Dermancentor variabilis*) and the western mountain or Rocky Mountain wood tick (*Dermancentor andersoni*). Rocky Mountain Spotted Fever occurs when these ticks inject a protozoan (*Rickettsia rickettsii*) into the dog while attached. The signs seen with this disease are:

- Weakness
- High fever (up to 105°F)
- Abdominal tenderness
- Water retention, especially in the legs

If you see any of the above signs call your veterinarian. Although there is no first aid as such for tick diseases, you may be able to prevent them by quickly checking your dog after a run through the woods. The tick may not have attached itself yet or may not have been attached long enough to cause an infection.

Use your fingertips to comb through the fur over the entire body, starting at the head and moving back. If you find a tick, remove it with tweezers (Figure 3-4 [Top]) or between your thumb and forefinger, pulling straight out (Figure 3-4 [Bottom]). Save it for your veterinarian to identify.

Bees, Wasps, Hornets and Ants

The stinging insects may pose a serious threat, especially if your dog is stung repeatedly or is hypersensitive to the venom (rare). The signs will vary with the location of the stings, with the number of stings and if your dog is sensitized:

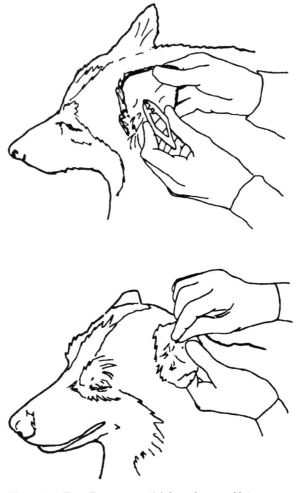

Figure 3-4: Top: To remove a tick from the ear with tweezer, steady the ear with one hand while grasping the tick with the tweezers where it is closest to the skin of the ear. Pull out evenly. **Bottom:** To remove a tick with your fingers, grasp it firmly between your thumb and index fingers where it is closest to the skin of the ear and pull straight out. If possible, use a tissue or cloth when pulling to avoid exposure to the tick. With your other hand, steady the ear.

- Pain and swelling in the area of the sting
- Difficulty breathing, if the stings were in the mouth
- Anaphylactic shock, if the dog is sensitized (see Chapter 3, Section 1)
- Shock, especially if there were multiple stings (see Chapter 1, Section 6)

First Aid

- If shock develops, transport your dog to a veterinarian immediately after calling ahead. Treat for shock in the car.
- Maintain an open airway if your dog has difficulty breathing (see Figure 3-1).
- If the leg is stung, make sure it remains below the level of the heart (see Figure 3-3 [Top left]).
- Remove the embedded stinger with tweezers (see Figure 3-5 [Top left]) or by scraping with a credit card (see Figure 3-5 [Top right]). Do not squeeze the stinger because the venom sac may burst.
- Apply cold packs to the swollen area (see Figure 3-5 [Bottom]). Do not use ice because it may freeze the skin.

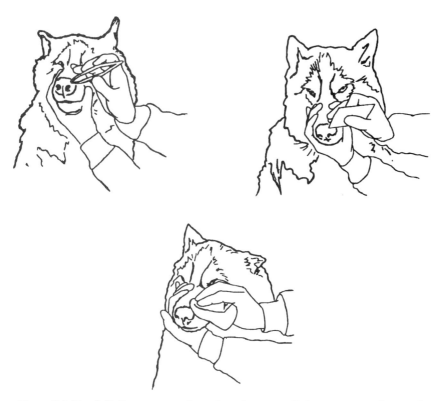

Figure 3-5: Top left: To remove a stinger from the nose with tweezers, restrain your dog with one hand around the lower part of the muzzle, while you use the tweezers with the other hand. **Top right:** To remove a stinger with a credit card, restrain your dog with one hand around the lower part of the muzzle. Scrape the surface of the nose with a credit card by rubbing it back and forth until the stinger is removed. **Bottom:** A cold pack is applied to the nose where the stinger was removed. Restrain your dog with one hand while holding the pack with the other.

- Apply a paste of either baking soda and water or Adolf's instant meat tenderizer and water to the area of the sting to neutralize the venom.

Spiders

Only two types of spiders are capable of causing severe injury to your dog: the female black widow (*Latrodectus mactans*) and the brown recluse (*Loxosceles reclusa*). The *black widow* is a shiny black spider, about ¾ inch in length, with a red hourglass-shaped spot on its underside. The *brown recluse* is a tawny to brown spider, about ½ inch in length, with long legs and a dark brown fiddle-shaped mark on its back. The black widow is found all over the United States, and the brown recluse is found mainly in the southern United States.

Black Widow

The signs of a black widow bite are:
- Severe pain at the site of the bite
- Muscle spasms
- Drooling
- Convulsions
- Difficulty breathing

First Aid

- Keep your dog still.
- If the leg has been bitten, keep it below the level of the heart (see Figure 3-3 [Top Left]).
- Watch for signs of allergic reactions (see Chapter 3, Section 1).
- Maintain an open airway (see Figure 3-1).

Brown Recluse

The signs associated with a brown recluse bite are:

- Initially, little pain or swelling associated with the bite will be present.
- After a few hours, a blister will form.
- After 1 to 2 weeks, an ulcer will develop.
- Fever.

No specific first aid is necessary; however, once you recognize the signs, it is important that the blister/ulcer be surgically removed as soon as possible so that the surrounding skin is not affected.

Scorpions

Two dangerous species of scorpions are present in the United States (Sculptured Centroides, *Centruroides sculpturatus* and *Vejovis spinigerus*) and both live in southern Arizona. The stinger which contains the venom is on the last segment of the scorpion's tail. The signs associated with scorpion stings are:

- Extreme pain, swelling and redness at the site of the sting
- Drooling
- Generalized weakness
- Paralysis
- Breathing difficulties

First Aid

- Apply cold packs on the sting, if possible. Do not use ice because it may freeze the skin.
- If your dog has breathing difficulties, maintain an open airway (see Chapter 1, Figure 3-1).

Lizards

Fortunately for dogs, lizards are not very aggressive and thus the number of biting incidences is low. Only two species of poisonous lizards are present in the United States: the Gila monster (*Heloderma suspectum*) and the Mexican beaded lizard (*Heloderma horridum*). Both are found in the southwestern United States. The signs associated with lizard bites are:

- Pain and swelling at the site of the bite
- Vomiting
- Shock

First Aid

- Remove the lizard, if it does not let go, by prying open the jaws with pliers.
- Flush the wound with plenty of water.
- Treat for shock (see Chapter 1, Section 6).

SECTION 4: BLOAT (GASTRIC TORSION)

Bloat occurs when the stomach of your dog fills with gas.

A gas-filled stomach may twist on itself, resulting in gastric torsion. As it twists on itself, it cuts off the blood supply, causes shock and, if not corrected quickly, results in death. The exact cause of this gas accumulation is not yet known, but some factors which may predispose your dog to this syndrome are:

- Large dogs with deep chests
- Overeating
- Overdrinking
- Exercising directly after eating

The signs of Bloat are:

- Drooling
- Restlessness
- Retching and foaming at the mouth
- Abdominal enlargement
- Abdominal pain
- Difficulty breathing
- Shock

First Aid

- Treat for shock during the trip to the clinic (see Chapter 1, Section 6).

SECTION 5: BURNS

Most cases of burns in dogs are due to *heat injury* from a heating pad, a heat lamp, a hot liquid spill or a flame, or *electrical injury* from biting an electrical cord; see Electric Shock, Section 8. *Chemical injury* from acid and alkali cleaners may also cause burns to the skin or mouth. If your dog becomes trapped in a burning building, smoke inhalation may cause burns to the lining of the breathing passages.

When severe, burns may cause shock, extreme pain and infection. The severity depends upon the age of the dog and the size, location and depth of the burn. Burns are considered serious when they affect very young or very old dogs, when they are spread over more than about 15% of the dog's body, when they occur on the head or joints or when the full

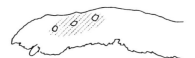
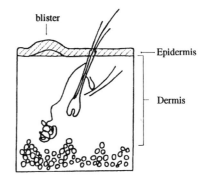

blister

Epidermis

Dermis

Figure 3-6: In a superficial or first degree burn, the injury to the skin is confined to the epidermis, which appears red and may blister. It will heal rapidly in most cases.

thickness of the skin is destroyed. The signs of a burn injury on the skin will mostly depend upon the depth of the burn. These are classified as:

Superficial or First Degree (see Figure 3-6)

Partial Thickness or Second Degree (see Figure 3-7)

Full Thickness or Third Degree (see Figure 3-8)

In general you should never put ice, oils or ointments on the burn, because ice can freeze the tissue and ointments are difficult to remove. You should also never use cotton or any material which has loose fibers to cover the burn, because fibers sticking to the burned tissue may be difficult to remove.

First aid methods will vary according to the type of burn; but for all burns other than a superficial heat burn, you should **see your veterinarian immediately.**

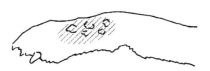
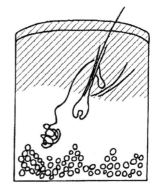

Figure 3-7: In a partial or second degree burn, the injury to the skin involves the epidermis and part of the dermis. Any blisters are broken and the surface initially appears red, wet and swollen. In a few days, it will dry to a tan-colored crust. This burn typically heals in about 2 weeks, if treated.

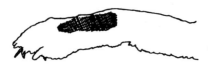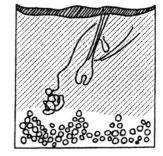

Figure 3-8: In a full or third degree burn, the injury extends to both layers of the skin and may extend under the skin. The surface appears blackened and there is no hair. It will heal very slowly with a scar unless a skin graft is done.

First Aid for Heat Burns

Superficial
- Clean gently with soap and water (see Figure 3-2 [Bottom left]).
- Apply cool compresses for 30 minutes (see Figure 3-9).
- Cover with a bandage (see Figure 3-2 [Bottom right] and Chapter 4, Section 2).

Partial or full thickness
- Treat shock.
- Cover with a loose bandage (see Figure 3-2 [Bottom right] and Chapter 4, Section 2).

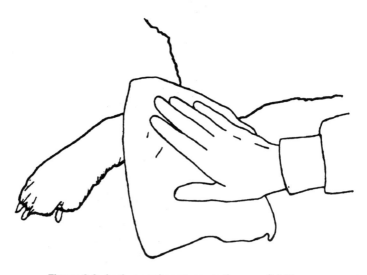

Figure 3-9: Apply a cool compress to the superficial burn.

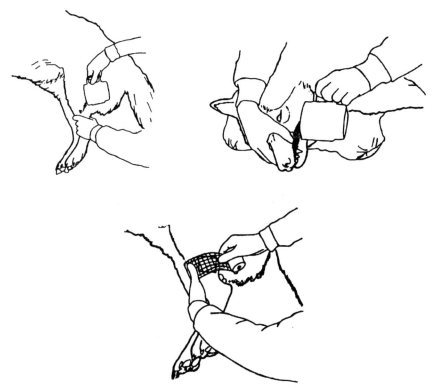

Figure 3-10: Top left: To flush a chemical burn, pour cool water from a cup or use a hose turned on low volume. **Top right:** To flush the mouth, lay your dog on his side, with neck and shoulders on a pillow so his head is lowered. With one hand, lift up his lip toward the back of his mouth. The other hand holds a cup or a slowly running hose. Flush large amounts of cool water through the mouth. **Bottom:** To cover a chemical burn, place a pad on the burn and cover loosely, first with gauze and then with adhesive (see Chapter 4, Section 2).

First Aid for Chemical Burns

- Remove contaminated collars or harnesses.
- Flush with cool running water for at least 20 minutes (see Figure 3-10 [Top left and right]).
- Cover with a bandage (see Figure 3-10 [Bottom], and Chapter 4, Section 2).

First Aid for Smoke Inhalation Burns

- Remove your dog from the source of smoke.
- Observe carefully for difficulty breathing, especially within the first 24 hours after the incident occurred.

SECTION 6: COMA

Coma occurs when your dog has a complete loss of consciousness, as in sleep, but has no response to pain.

It can be caused by an underlying disease in many different organs: brain, heart, kidney, liver, lung and pancreas. It may also be caused by certain drugs, poisons, temperature extremes, shock and infections. Because there are so many different causes, some of which may cause death within a very short period of time, it is very important to recognize the signs and provide first aid while on the way to your veterinarian. The two major signs of coma are:

- Sleep-like appearance
- No response to pain

First Aid

- Keep an airway open at all times.
- Monitor and provide CPR, if necessary, until your dog can be examined.

SECTION 7: DIABETIC EMERGENCIES

These emergencies can occur when either too much insulin (causing low blood sugar) or too little insulin (causing high blood sugar) is given when treating a diabetic dog. They are both considered major emergencies because, if untreated, they can lead to coma and death over a short period of time. In both cases, your veterinarian should be notified immediately.

Too Much Insulin

The signs begin about 3 to 7 hours after the last dose of insulin and include:

- Weakness
- Fatigue
- Seizures
- Coma

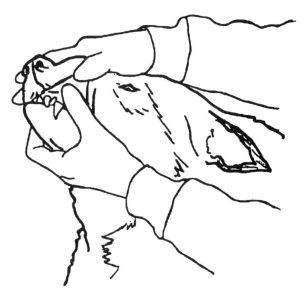

Figure 3-11: To rub a glucose-containing syrup on your dog's gums, place one hand over your dog's muzzle and lift up the lip with your thumb. Pour some syrup on the thumb of your other hand and rub this into the gums.

First Aid

- Keep a bottle of a glucose-containing syrup (for example, Karo syrup) available in your home and get an appropriate dosage from your veterinarian in case you need to use it.
- If convulsions start, do not attempt to pour the syrup into your dog's mouth, as he will choke. Instead, give the syrup as shown in Figure 3-11.

Too Little Insulin

If you have forgotten to give your dog his insulin injection or give him too little, you may notice the following signs:

- Depression
- Weakness
- Sweet, fruity smell to the breath
- Vomiting
- Coma

First Aid

- Give your dog his normal dose of insulin immediately.

NOTE: **If your dog is not being treated for diabetes and is showing the signs described above, he may have diabetes. Have him examined by your veterinarian.**

SECTION 8: ELECTRIC SHOCK

In most cases, electric shock in dogs is due to chewing on an electric cord. A typical household AC outlet has a frequency of 60 Hz. When your dog contacts an exposed wire, the dog's heart will beat erratically and the lungs will fill with fluid. The signs will be:

- Difficulty breathing
- Burns in and around the mouth
- Loss of consciousness
- Heart stops

First Aid

- If your dog still has the electric cord in his mouth, pull the plug out before providing first aid.
- Provide CPR support as needed.
- Treat burns around the mouth if possible with cool compresses (not ice; see Figure 3-12).
- Monitor respiration and pulse rates often, especially during the first 12 hours following the accident.

SECTION 9: POISONING

Dogs may be poisoned by many substances in our environment. The causes range from common household items such as insecticides, cleaning solutions and antifreeze to the seeds, bark and leaves of many different plants. Dogs may even be poisoned by mouthing or biting certain toads and salamanders.

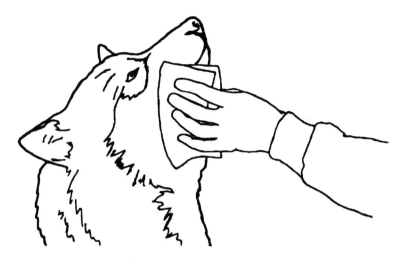

Figure 3-12: To treat burns around the mouth, hold a cool compress on the injured area.

It is important to remember that all drugs, even common household medicines, may cause poisoning in your dog. Always check with your veterinarian *before* giving your dog any drug.

You may have a clue as to what your dog ingested by seeing bits of chewed plant, bottles of cleaning solution chewed open and medicine bottles broken open with some or most of the pills gone. The signs your dog will show from any type of poison will mostly depend on the quantity ingested, but in general you should suspect that your dog has been poisoned if you see the following signs occur *suddenly:*

- Drooling
- Vomiting
- Fatigue
- Convulsions

Table 3-2 lists the common poisons, their major sources and the first aid required when these poisons are ingested. For cases of external poisoning (for example, a spill on the fur or overdose of flea powder) involving the chemicals listed in Table 3-2, please see General First Aid below. Table 3-3 details plant poisoning by common name/toxic part, the signs and first aid. Poisonings from toads and salamanders are discussed following the General First Aid section.

TABLE 3-2 Common Poisons

Poison	Source	First Aid
Acids	cleaning solutions etching solutions household chlorine bleach	1. DO NOT INDUCE VOMITING. 2. Rinse out mouth with water. 3. Give 1 to 2 tablespoons of cooking oil or mineral oil, once.
Alkalis	ammonia washing powders paint removers laundry detergents	1. DO NOT INDUCE VOMITING. 2. Rinse out mouth with water. 3. Give 1 to 2 tablespoons of cooking oil or mineral oil, once.
Arsenic	insecticides herbicides paint	1. Induce vomiting. 2. Give activated charcoal. *Antidote available* *from veterinarian*
Carbamates	insecticides: Carbaryl® Sevin® Propoxur®	1. Induce vomiting. 2. Give activated charcoal. *Antidote available* *from veterinarian*
Carbon monoxide	exhaust fumes	1. Remove the dog from the source of fumes. 2. Give CPR, if necessary. 3. Monitor closely for 48 hours.
Drugs (human)	aspirin acetaminophen (Tylenol)®	1. Induce vomiting. 2. Give activated charcoal. *Antidote available* *from veterinarian*
Ethylene glycol	antifreeze	1. Induce vomiting. 2. Give activated charcoal. *Antidote available* *from veterinarian*
Lead	insecticides paint ceramics linoleum golf balls	1. Induce vomiting. 2. Give activated charcoal. *Antidote available* *from veterinarian*

Metaldehyde	rodenticide snail bait	1. Induce vomiting. 2. Give activated charcoal.
Organophosphates	insecticides: Dichlorvos® Fenthion® Parathion® Ronnel® Trichlorfon®	1. Induce vomiting. 2. Give activated charcoal. *Antidote available from veterinarian*
Petroleum distillates	motor oil gasoline turpentine paint paint thinner paint remover lighter fluid kerosene	1. DO NOT INDUCE VOMITING. 2. Give 1 to 2 tablespoons of cooking oil or mineral oil, once.
Phenol	disinfectants (Lysol®) fungicides herbicides wood preservatives photographic developers	1. Induce vomiting. 2. Give activated charcoal.
Strychnine	rodenticides	1. Induce vomiting only if no there are no signs of breathing difficulty. 2. Give activated charcoal.
Vitamin D_3	rodenticides	1. Induce vomiting. 2. Give activated charcoal. 3. Keep dog out of sunlight. *Antidote available from veterinarian*
Warfarin	rodenticide	1. Induce vomiting. 2. Give activated charcoal. *Antidote available from veterinarian*

TABLE 3-3 Cont.

Common Name/Toxic Part	Symptoms	First Aid
azalea, rhododendron/*leaf*	repeated swallowing, excess saliva	1. Induce vomiting. 2. Give activated charcoal.
tulip, daffodil, amaryllis, iris/*bulb*	depression, vomiting	1. Induce vomiting. 2. Give activated charcoal.
castor bean, precatory bean/*bean*	fever, profuse bloody diarrhea	1. Induce vomiting. 2. Give activated charcoal. 3. Monitor for signs of shock.
English ivy/*fruit*	intense thirst, vomiting, diarrhea, may die within 1–2 days	1. Induce vomiting. 2. Give activated charcoal.
mistletoe/*berries*	vomiting, diarrhea	1. Induce vomiting. 2. Give activated charcoal.
mushroom poisoning (family: *Amanifaceae*)/*cap*	vomiting, diarrhea, muscle spasms	1. Induce vomiting. 2. Give activated charcoal.
black nightshade, Jerusalem cherry, climbing nightshade/*berries*	vomiting, bloody diarrhea, trembling, weakness	1. Induce vomiting. 2. Give activated charcoal.
English walnuts, black walnuts/*hulls*	vomiting, diarrhea, convulsions	1. Induce vomiting. 2. Give activated charcoal.
snow-on-the-mountain, crown-of-thorns, tinsel tree-milk bush, poinsettia/*irritant sap in leaves*	inflammation to skin and eye, vomiting, diarrhea	1. Induce vomiting. 2. Give activated charcoal.
dumb cane, philodendron, elephant ears, skunk cabbage/*leaves*	swelling of the tongue and throat, difficulty breathing	1. Keep airway open. 2. CPR if necessary.

		3. DO NOT INDUCE VOMITING.
stinging nettle, bull nettles, nettle spurge/*hair all over plant*	burning in mouth, muscle weakness, slow and irregular heartbeat	1. Keep dog quiet. 2. DO NOT INDUCE VOMITING.
tobacco/*leaves*	vomiting, diarrhea, difficulty breathing, staggering, weakness	1. Induce vomiting. 2. Give activated charcoal. 3. Keep airway open. 4. Give CPR if necessary.
Japanese yew/*needles, bark, seed*	muscular weakness, difficulty breathing	1. Induce vomiting. 2. Give activated charcoal. 3. Keep airway open. 4. Give CPR if necessary.
oleander (very toxic)/*leaf, bark, stems;* lily of the valley/*bulb;* purple foxglove/*all parts*	depression, bloody diarrhea, fast or slow heart beat	1. Induce vomiting. 2. Give activated charcoal.
bitter cherry, choke cherry, wild black cherry, apricot, almond, apple/*seeds*	cyanide poisoning: bright red gums, involuntary urination and defecation, labored breathing, convulsions, frothing at the mouth, coma	1. Induce vomiting. 2. Give activated charcoal. *Antidote available*
jimsonweed/*seeds*	dry red skin, fever, convulsions	1. Induce vomiting. 2. Give activated charcoal.
burdock/*hooked barbs of florets*	lacerated eyes, ears, nose, trachea, bronchus	1. Clean & treat wounds (C. 4, S. 1). 2. Bandage (C. 4, S. 2).

Common Name/Toxic Part	Symptoms	First Aid
burdock *(cont.)*		3. Keep airway open. 4. CPR if necessary.
rose, blackberry, dewberry/*hooked barbs of stems*	punctures and lacerations of eye, mouth, skin and feet	1. Clean & treat wounds (C. 4, S. 1). 2. Bandage (C. 4, S. 2).
quince, hawthorn, Osage orange/*heavy spines on stems*	stab wounds of eye, skin, feet and legs	1. Clean & treat wounds (C. 4, S. 1). 2. Bandage (C. 4, S. 2).
honey locust/*pronged spines*	eye lacerations and puncture wounds of skin	1. Clean & treat wounds (C. 4, S. 1). 2. Bandage (C. 4, S. 2).
cactus/*sharp spines of leaf* grasses (foxtail, wild barley, june grass, ripgut grass)/*awns, barbs, fragmented seed heads*	multiple punctures with migrating spine fragments barbs penetrate and migrate into ear canal, air passages, under skin and into body cavities	1. Clean & treat wounds (C. 4, S. 1). 2. Bandage (C. 4, S. 2). 3. Remove by clipping all spines, awns, barbs or seed heads which are caught in the hair. 4. All migrating parts must be removed surgically.

C = Chapter
S = Section

General First Aid

1. If your dog is unconscious, check the airway, breathing and circulation and perform CPR as necessary.
2. Call your veterinarian and be able to tell what the poison is, what the active ingredients are (if you know them), how much was taken, when it was taken and what signs your dog is showing.
3. If your veterinarian cannot be reached, call the National Animal Poison Control Center at one of the following numbers:
   - 1-900-680-0000
   - 1-800-548-2423

   These numbers are answered 24 hours per day, 7 days per week. There is a charge for these services.
4. Take the following steps for poison ingested within the past 2 hours:
   - If your dog is conscious and you know the poison is *not* a petroleum product, cleaning solution or a strong acid or alkali, induce vomiting using either 3% hydrogen peroxide *at a dosage of 1 to 2 teaspoons by mouth every 15 minutes until vomiting occurs* or syrup of ipecac *at a dosage of 2 to 3 teaspoons by mouth given once;* see Appendix 2, Figure A-1 [left].
   - Inspect the vomit and save a sample for your veterinarian.
   - Once vomiting has occurred, activated charcoal at a dosage of 1 to 2 teaspoons of powder mixed to a slurry with water given by mouth once may be given to absorb the remaining toxin. *Do not* use activated charcoal if vomiting has not occurred.
5. With the exception of paint, tar, motor oil and similar substances, poisons which are not taken internally and remain on the outside of your dog can be removed by following these steps:
   - Flush the area with large amounts of water for at least 5 minutes.
   - Wear gloves and wash your dog with mild soap and water.
6. To remove paint, tar or motor oil from the fur or skin of your dog:
   - Wearing gloves, rub in large amounts of mineral oil or vegetable oil before the poisons harden.
   - After the poisons become loosened, bathe your dog in warm water made soapy with a mild dishwashing liquid.
   - Rinse well, repeat if necessary.
   - In severe cases, dust your dog with cornmeal, cornstarch or flour after you have rubbed in the mineral oil. This will help

to remove more of the toxin. To remove, comb or brush your dog and bathe in warm, soapy water.
- Remember not to use turpentine, paint thinner or mineral spirits to remove these substances.

Toads and Salamanders

As mentioned above, dogs become poisoned by biting or mouthing certain toads and salamanders. Puppies are the most susceptible to severe reactions.

Toads

Two species of toads in the United States can be poisonous to dogs: Colorado River toads (*Bufo alvarius*) and marine toads (*Bufo marinus*). The Colorado River toads are found in the Southwest, while the marine toads are found in Florida.

The signs seen in toad poisoning occur rapidly and are:

- Profuse salivation
- Difficulty breathing
- Convulsions
- Prostration

First Aid

- Flush mouth with large quantities of water (see Figure 3-10 [Top right]).
- Maintain an open airway (see Figure 3-1).
- Give CPR, if necessary (see Chapter 1, Section 3).

Salamanders

The California newt (*Taricha torosa*) is the only species of poisonous salamander in the United States. It is found in California.

The signs are:

- Weakness and incoordination
- Vomiting and diarrhea (puppies only)
- Paralysis

First Aid

- Dogs usually recover quickly without treatment.
- You can help your dog recover more quickly by washing his mouth with large quantities of water (see Figure 3-10 [Top right]).

SECTION 10: SEIZURES

Seizures occur when there is a sudden disturbance in brain function.

If this disturbance spreads to a specific area of the brain, the seizure is said to be partial; if it spreads to a broad area of the brain, the seizure is said to be generalized. Seizures may be caused by a brain tumor, lack of oxygen, low blood sugar, liver disease, viruses or poisons. Sometimes, however, they have no known cause and are called idiopathic. *If the seizures recur, the condition is known as epilepsy.*

Partial Seizures

The signs seen will depend upon the type of seizure. If the seizure is partial, you might see either:

- Convulsions limited to a specific area of the body (for example, the right front leg) or
- Specific behavioral changes such as drooling and licking, sudden blindness or eating nonfood items such as drapes, furniture, etc.

Generalized Seizures

The most common generalized seizure is the *grand mal* and consists of *4 stages:*

- *Aura*: This is the time just before the seizure. Your dog will be restless and anxious and may want to be close to you. This will last 1 to 2 minutes.
- *Prodome*: This is the stage at which your dog loses consciousness; it will last for 1 to 2 seconds.
- *Ictus*: In this stage, your dog will remain unconscious and will have convulsions accompanied by urination, defecation, drooling and dilated pupils. This stage lasts from a few seconds to a few minutes.

- *Postictal*: At this stage, your dog will regain consciousness and will show blindness, confusion and weakness. It can last from a few hours to a few days.

The petit mal *seizure is another type of generalized seizure.* It is rare in dogs, but the signs are:

- Sudden loss of consciousness and muscle tone without convulsions
- Lasts only a few seconds

First Aid

- If you notice the aura stage, immediately engage your dog in an activity which he likes (for example, chasing a ball). This may prevent him from having a seizure.
- If convulsions start, make sure the ground is smooth and clear of all objects which he may hit during the seizure.
- **Do not** attempt to hold your dog's mouth open or shut.
- Keep other dogs away from the seizuring dog, as they may attack him while he is seizuring.
- After the convulsions, keep your dog confined and monitor the temperature, breathing and pulse (see Chapter 1, Section 1).
- Keep a good record of all seizures your dog has had. Note the time of day and date, the number of hours after a meal and anything unusual which coincided with the event. This will help your veterinarian in trying to find a cause and recommend treatment.
- You should notify your veterinarian immediately if:
  a. The seizures occur one after another, with little or no period of rest in between. This condition is called *status epilepticus* and is a major emergency.
  b. The seizure lasts for more than a few minutes.

SECTION 11: TEMPERATURE EXTREMES

Dogs exposed to very high or very low environmental temperatures may suffer drastic changes in their own body temperatures.

How much the body temperature changes will greatly depend on the extent and duration of the exposure as well as the age and physical condition of the dog. It is important to note that both temperature extremes can cause seizures, coma and death.

High Temperatures

Heat stroke, eclampsia and seizure disorders can all cause your dog's body temperature to be very high (above 105°F).

Heat Stroke

Heat stroke most often occurs when dogs are confined during hot weather. Some of the initial signs are:

- Panting
- Increased pulse
- Bright red gums
- High body temperature (105-110°F)

Later the signs will be:

- Stupor
- Shock
- Pale gums
- Vomiting
- Diarrhea

Finally, the signs are:

- Coma
- No breathing

First Aid

- Move your dog to a cool, ventilated area.
- Give CPR, if necessary.
- Give your dog a cold or ice water bath.
- Take a rectal temperature every 10 minutes.
- Stop the bath when the temperature reaches 103°F.
- Treat for shock.
- Do not give aspirin.

Eclampsia and Seizures

In these conditions, body temperatures become very high due to heat produced through muscle movement. *Eclampsia* refers to the muscle tremors which may occur in the female dog after whelping. In seizures, especially those which are clustered together or prolonged, the muscle action during the convulsions can cause high body temperatures (see Seizures, Section 10).

First Aid

- Take the temperature. In a case of eclampsia, first remove the puppies from the mother. In a case of seizures, wait until your dog has stopped having convulsions before taking the temperature.
- If the temperature is above 105°F, start cold or ice water baths as for heat stroke.
- Take a rectal temperature every 10 minutes.
- Stop the bath when the temperature reaches 103°F.

Low Temperatures

Exposure to extremely cold weather can produce generalized body chilling to temperatures of 77 to 95°F (and sometimes lower). This condition is called *hypothermia*. Cold exposure may also produce frostbite, which is a freezing of small areas of the body. Sometimes, both hypothermia and frostbite occur together.

Hypothermia

The major signs seen in hypothermia are:

- Low body temperatures (below 95°F)
- Very slow pulse rate
- Very slow breathing rate
- Seizures
- Coma

First Aid

- Give your dog a warm water bath or wrap him in blankets in a warm room. Use blankets which have been warmed in a dryer for a few minutes.
- Take a rectal temperature every 10 minutes.
- Stop the bath when the temperature reaches 101°F.
- Beware of hot water bottles and electric blankets as these may burn the skin.

Frostbite

Mild cases of frostbite have the following signs:

- Skin will first appear pale.
- Skin later becomes red, hot, painful and swollen.
- Skin will eventually return to normal but will always be extra sensitive.

Severe cases of frostbite have the following signs:

- Skin stays cold and starts to shrivel.
- Skin will eventually slough, leaving behind a raw wound.

First Aid

Mild frostbite
- Warm the frostbitten area rapidly with a water bath between 105-108°F for about 15 minutes.
- Cover with a loose bandage (see Chapter 4, Section 2).
- Do not rub the skin.

Severe frostbite
- Treat as mild frostbite.
- Tissue which is devitalized must be removed by your veterinarian.

SECTION 12: URINARY TRACT BLOCKAGE

Blockage of the urinary tract occurs mostly in male dogs because their urethras, which lead from the bladder to the outside, are quite narrow and long.

Most often, blockage is caused by uroliths, which are small stones composed of mineral salts. These stones are formed in the bladder, become caught in the urethra and prevent urine from leaving the bladder. The major signs are:

- Straining to urinate
- Bloody urine
- Dehydration
- Shock

First Aid

- If you see the signs described above, have your dog examined immediately.
- Treat for shock (see Chapter 1, Section 6).

SECTION 13: VOMITING AND DIARRHEA

Vomiting and diarrhea are considered together because they share many of the same causes and signs; the first aid for the two conditions is nearly identical.

Vomiting

A change in diet (new food or eating garbage), intestinal worms, contagious viral diseases (parvovirus, distemper and coronavirus) and a foreign object in the stomach or intestine are some of the major causes of vomiting in dogs of all ages.

In puppies, sudden vomiting may also be caused by an *intussusception*, which occurs when one part of the intestine pushes into the inside of another part. In more mature dogs, any of the following may also cause vomiting: inflammation of the pancreas, liver disease, kidney disease, ulcers, poisons or gastrointestinal tumors. The signs that your dog may be about to vomit are:

- Drooling
- Excessive swallowing
- Abdominal contractions (retching)
- Pacing and restlessness

Vomiting may then cause:

- Weakness
- Dehydration
- Shock (if vomiting is severe)

Diarrhea

Diarrhea occurs when the frequency and the fluid content of the bowel movement are increased. The major causes of diarrhea are abrupt diet changes, intestinal worms, contagious viral diseases (parvovirus,

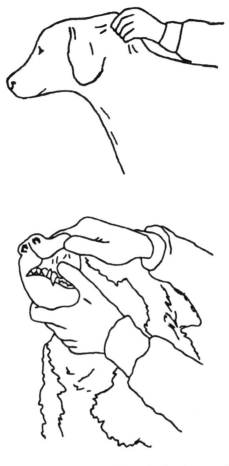

Figure 3-13: Top: To check if your dog has become dehydrated from vomiting and diarrhea, pick up the skin at the back of the neck between your thumb and forefinger and then let it go. It will assume its normal position immediately in a hydrated dog. The longer it takes to go down, the more dehydrated your dog is. **Bottom:** You can also check for dehydration by touching your dog's gums. To do this, put one hand on the top of your dog's muzzle, lifting up the lip. With the thumb of your other hand, touch the gums. If they feel tacky or dry, your dog is dehydrated.

distemper and coronavirus), drugs (antibiotics and anticancer drugs), stress and poisons. The signs seen with diarrhea are the same as vomiting:

- Weakness
- Dehydration
- Shock (if diarrhea is severe)

First Aid

- First check to see if your dog is dehydrated (see Figure 3-13).
- If your dog is dehydrated, notify you veterinarian at once as this condition could easily lead to shock.
- If your dog is not dehydrated and is vomiting, confine him and withhold food and water for 12-24 hours. You can offer ice cubes for your dog to lick.
- If your dog is not dehydrated and has diarrhea but is not vomiting, confine him and withhold food for 12-24 hours. You can offer small amounts of water during this time.
- Note what the vomit/diarrhea looks like and save some in an airtight container in your refrigerator for your veterinarian to examine.
- If your dog has had no vomiting/diarrhea after 12-24 hours, you can offer 1 to 2 tablespoons of broth or baby food every 3 hours. If your dog continues without vomiting/diarrhea, increase these foods and gradually introduce the standard fare over the next 2 to 3 days.
- Notify your veterinarian in any of the following situations: if vomiting/diarrhea persists during the 12-24 hours when food and water are restricted, if vomiting/diarrhea begins again with eating and drinking, if you find blood in the vomit/diarrhea, or if shock develops (see Chapter 1, Section 6).
- Treat for shock if necessary (see Chapter 1, Section 6).

SUMMARY

In summary, the emergencies listed in this chapter require action within a few minutes to a few hours if your dog is not to suffer severe illness or loss of life. An important first step is being able to recognize the signs of each emergency. Often, if the emergency is recognized sufficiently early and the proper steps are taken, you may be able to reduce the complications associated with the emergency and, in so doing, save your dog's life.

4

General Aid Techniques

WOUNDS AND FRACTURES accompany most injuries, especially traumatic ones. Since wounds may become infected quickly, it is important to know how to clean and bandage them, even before you arrive at the emergency clinic. If possible, fractures should be splinted to reduce swelling and lessen the chances of further injury during transport.

This chapter will cover wounds and wound care including how to apply specific bandages in different emergency situations. A description of the different classes of fractures is provided as well as how to recognize and treat fractures. Finally, dislocations, sprains and strains are defined and the first aid for these conditions is discussed.

SECTION 1: WOUNDS

The two basic classes of wounds are: *closed* (when the skin is not broken) and *open* (when the skin is broken). This section will describe and illustrate general wound care and then discuss the many different types of open wounds which exist and specific first aid where it is pertinent.

Wound Care

Closed Wounds

A closed wound is also known as a bruise or contusion. It may occur in mild trauma and alongside open wounds in severe trauma. The signs include:

- Swelling
- Pain
- Discoloration of the injured area due to bleeding under the skin

First Aid

- Within a few hours of the injury, apply cool compresses (not ice) to the wound.
- After 24 hours, use warm compresses.
- Look for signs of other injuries, especially if your dog was hit by a car.

Open Wounds

In open wounds, underlying tissues are exposed since the skin has been broken. These wounds must be treated immediately to avoid infection, preferably within the first six hours.

First Aid for Wounds with Severe Bleeding

- Stop the bleeding (see Chapter 1, Section 6).
- Bandage the wound (see Section 2 of this chapter). Remember to incorporate the blood-soaked pad into the bandage, as removing the pad would disturb clot formation.
- Treat for shock (see Chapter 1, Section 6).

First Aid for Wounds Without Severe Bleeding

- Wash your hands.
- Put first aid materials on a clean blanket or towel within easy reach.
- Do not cough or breathe over the wound and do not touch it unless necessary.
- If you are using sterile pads or dressings, handle only the edges.

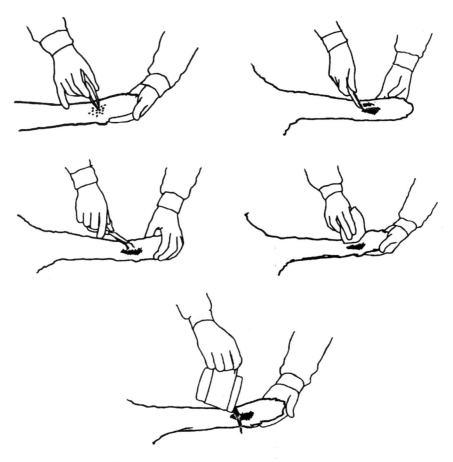

Figure 4-1: Top left: Removing gravel from the wound with tweezers. **Top right:** Combing mud or blood out of the fur surrounding the wound. Comb away from the wound. **Middle left:** Clipping the hair surrounding the wound with scissors. **Middle right:** Use a clean cloth with soap and water to clean the skin surrounding the wound. Clean from the edge of the wound outward. **Bottom:** To clean the wound itself, pour plenty of fresh, cool water over it.

- Use tweezers to remove gravel and splinters from the wound itself (see Figure 4-1 [Top left]).
- If mud- or blood-soaked hair is on the skin surrounding the wound, attempt to remove this by wetting it or by combing it away from the wound (see Figure 4-1 [Top right]).
- Using scissors which have been lubricated with petroleum jelly on the blades, clip the hair surrounding the wound (see Figure 4-1 [Middle left]).
- Clean the skin surrounding the wound with soap and warm water. Use cotton balls or a washcloth and clean away from the wound (see Figure 4-1 [Middle right]).

- Use a water pik or plenty of cool, clean water poured from a bottle or cup to clean the wound (see Figure 4-1 [Bottom]). Use only water; do not use soap, detergent or hydrogen peroxide.
- Bandage the wound (see Section 2).

Infected Wounds

If a wound becomes infected, you will see the following signs:

- The wound will be painful, red, swollen and warm.
- Lameness, if the infection is on the leg.
- Pus, either draining from the wound or collected under the bandage.
- Fever, weakness and decreased appetite.
- Signs of tetanus if the wound was contaminated with the bacteria, *Clostridium tetani* (see tetanus, below).

First Aid

- Change the bandage and rinse all pus away with water.
- Have your dog examined as soon as possible.

Tetanus

Tetanus is caused by bacteria, *Clostridium tetani*, which live in the soil and the feces of various animals (including man). The bacteria grow very well and rapidly in deep puncture wounds. The signs may develop 1 to 2 weeks after your dog was wounded and are:

- Ears standing straight up
- General stiffness and paralysis
- Inability to stand
- Hypersensitivity to light and noise in the environment

First Aid

- If your dog does incur a puncture wound which you suspect may have been contaminated with soil or feces, notify your veterinarian immediately.
- If your dog develops signs of tetanus, keep her in a dark, quiet environment until she can be treated.

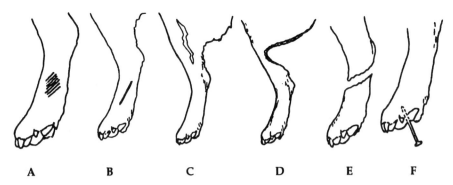

Figure 4-2: A. Abrasion. An abrasion occurs when the skin is scraped by a hard surface; little bleeding is observed. **B.** Incision. A cut from a sharp object with smooth, straight edges (such as a piece of broken glass, razor blade or a knife) can cause an incision. Heavy bleeding may be present along with possible damage to nerves and muscles. **C.** Laceration. A laceration occurs when the skin is cut by an object with sharp irregular edges. A bite wound is a good example of a laceration. The tissue damage can be very great. **D.** Avulsion. Avulsions occur when a body part is torn from the body, but not completely separated as may occur in trap wounds and automobile accidents. **E.** Amputation. Amputations occur when a body part, usually a leg, becomes severed from the rest of the body, as with lawn mower and chain saw accidents. **F.** Puncture. Pointed objects such as teeth, bullets, nails, pins, arrows, splinters and porcupine quills can cause puncture wounds. Because these wounds are difficult to clean, infections may easily occur, including tetanus (see above).

- If you have a dog which does search and rescue or police work, see your veterinarian about getting an immunization for tetanus.

Types of Open Wounds

The types of open wounds which you are likely to encounter are described and illustrated in Figure 4-2. While nearly all of these wounds are treated by following the first aid procedures discussed above, in some cases (e.g., puncture wounds) additional methods are required.

Specific first aid procedures for different types of puncture wounds are given below:

First Aid for Splinters

- Wash the skin surface with mild soap and water.
- Sterilize tweezers by boiling for 5 minutes or heating the tips over a flame. Wipe off the black carbon coating with a sterile pad.
- Remove the splinter (see Figure 4-3).
- Once the splinter is removed, wash the area again with soap and water. If the splinter had soil or dirt on it, notify your veterinarian of this fact as your dog may require tetanus antitoxin.

103

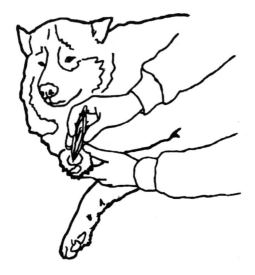

Figure 4-3: To remove a splinter, first loosen the skin surrounding the splinter with the end of the tweezers and then pull the splinter straight out.

- If the splinter breaks or is too deeply lodged to remove, cover it with a sterile pad or clean cloth and wrap it lightly with adhesive tape. Have your veterinarian remove it as soon as possible.

First Aid for Porcupine Quills

- If possible, have your veterinarian remove the quills. A veterinarian will likely do this with anesthesia and it will be less painful for your dog.
- If you cannot see your veterinarian, you can remove the quills with a needlenose or long nose pliers (see Figure 4-4).

First Aid for Arrow Impalement

- Do not remove the arrow as you may cause more damage by pulling it out.
- Cut the arrow about 2 inches from your dog's body and keep the dog confined until the arrow can be removed by your veterinarian.

SECTION 2: BANDAGING

This section will emphasize proper bandaging technique. We will first describe and illustrate the three main parts of a bandage and then elaborate on how to bandage specific parts of the body for the most

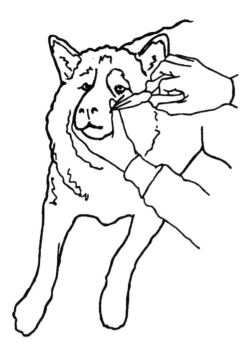

Figure 4-4: To remove a porcupine quill, pull the quill out following the angle of the shaft.

common emergencies. How best to keep the bandage on your dog (including the use of an Elizabethan collar) is also discussed.

Purpose

There are four good reasons to bandage a wound:

1. To keep the wound from becoming more contaminated
2. To protect it from further trauma, including self-mutilation
3. To keep it moist
4. To absorb blood seeping from the wound

General Technique

A simple bandage is made up of three layers: a pad, gauze and adhesive tape. In certain bandages, other materials must be added; these are discussed below under specific bandages.

Pad

This is the first layer of the bandage and is the part which comes into direct contact with the wound. In general, nonstick pads are better as they will not disturb any healing which takes place. Sterile pads are preferable to nonsterile pads, but most importantly, you should use something which is absorbent, clean and dust-free, even if it is a washcloth or piece of towel.

It is not necessary to put ointment on the pad before you place it over the wound. If you want to use an ointment, use Neosporin® or Bacitracin. *Do not use petroleum jelly* because it is not water soluble and therefore is very difficult to clean off the wound. Never put ointment on

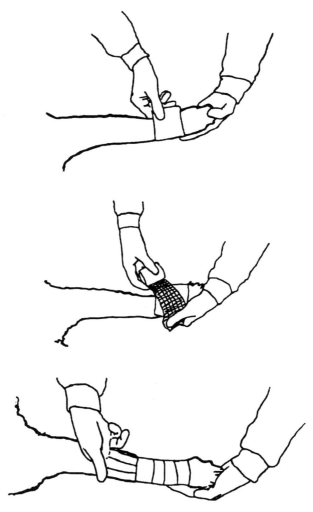

Figure 4-5: Top: Place the pad over the cleaned wound. **Middle:** Wrap the gauze over the pad. **Bottom:** Wrap the adhesive tape over the gauze. Two fingers should be able to fit between the bandage and the skin.

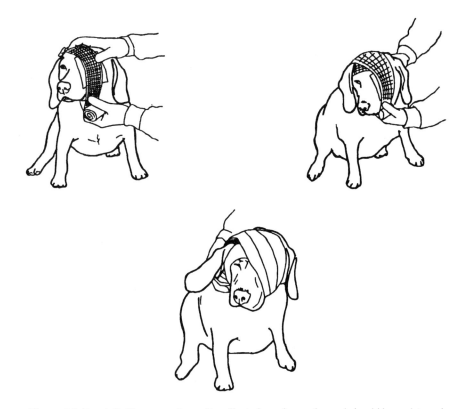

Figure 4-6: Top left: Place a pad over the affected eye (NOTE: the pad should be moistened with sterile saline or cool water before being placed against a prolapsed eye). Gauze is wrapped over the pad, starting at the top of the head in front of the ear opposite the affected eye. **Top right:** The gauze is continued under the chin and around the head, this time going behind the ear opposite the affected eye. Continue wrapping in this fashion, alternating the gauze in front of and behind the ear opposite the affected eye. **Bottom:** Cover the gauze with adhesive tape in the same manner as the gauze was applied.

the pad when bandaging deep wounds, open fractures or burns because these wounds are extremely difficult to clean once ointment has been applied. Place the pad over the cleaned wound (see Wounds, Section 1 and Figure 4-5 [Top]).

Gauze

The middle layer is made up of gauze. It is not advisable to use elastic or stretch gauze. Although it is easier to apply, it is also easier to wrap too tightly, increasing the chances of cutting off the circulation, causing swelling and cool and bluish-colored skin. The gauze is rolled over the pad so it is secure but not too tight (see Figure 4-5 [Middle]). As you roll, you should try to overlap the gauze by about ⅓ of its width.

107

Adhesive Tape

The outer layer consists of adhesive tape which holds the bandage down. Elastic adhesive may cause the same problem as elastic gauze. The adhesive tape should be applied in the same manner as the gauze (see Figure 4-5 [Bottom]), catching bits of hair at the top edge and bottom edge of the bandage.

To ensure that the bandage was not put on too tightly, you should always be able to fit two fingers between the bandage and the skin (see Figure 4-5 [Bottom]). This must be done for all bandages you apply. The bandage should be changed daily unless your veterinarian advises otherwise.

Specific Bandages

Eye

For eye injuries involving nonpenetrating foreign objects, trauma to the eye surface and lids and prolapse of the eye, see Figure 4-6.

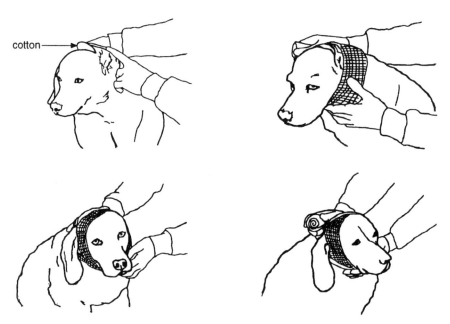

Figure 4-7: Top left: Place a pad against the cleaned wound and a piece of roll cotton between the ear and the head. **Top right:** Wrap the gauze over the ear so that the injured ear lies on top of the head. **Bottom left:** Wrap the gauze around the head, alternately in front of and behind the normal ear. **Bottom right:** Adhesive tape covers the gauze and is applied in the same manner as the gauze.

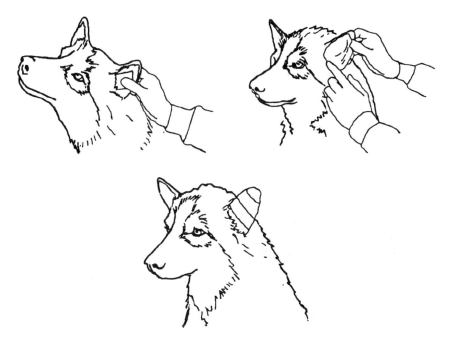

Figure 4-8: Top left: Place a pad against the cleaned wound. **Top right:** Mold a piece of cotton to fit into the ear. **Bottom:** Secure the molded cotton with short strips of adhesive tape going from the edge of the ear across the cotton to the other edge. When the bandage is finished, the cotton should be completely covered with the tape.

Ear

> For wounds to a pendulous ear, see Figure 4-7.
> For wounds to an erect ear, see Figure 4-8.

Neck

> For any wounds to the neck, see Figure 4-9.

Chest/Abdomen

> For any wounds of the chest or abdomen, see Figure 4-10.

Rump

> For all wounds of the rump, see Figure 4-11.

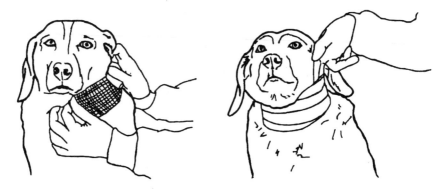

Figure 4-9: Left: Place a pad over the cleaned wound and wrap gauze over the pad with as little tension as possible. **Right:** Cover the gauze with adhesive tape making sure that two fingers can fit easily between the bandage and the neck. Your dog should not have any difficulty breathing while the bandage is on.

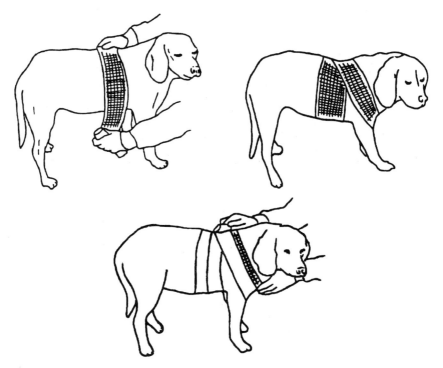

Figure 4-10: Top left: Place a pad against the wound (NOTE: for chest wounds, wet the pad with sterile saline or cool water and apply at the end of an exhalation) and cover with gauze starting at the top of the back. **Top right:** To make sure the gauze doesn't slip backward, wrap the gauze around the trunk alternating in front of and behind the foreleg on the same side as the wound. **Bottom:** Cover the gauze with adhesive tape in the same manner as the gauze was applied. To keep the bandage more secure, catch a small amount of fur at the edges of the bandage.

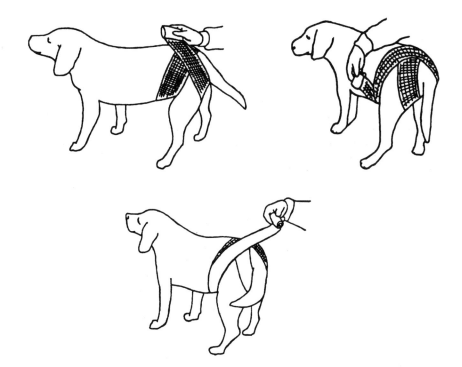

Figure 4-11: Top left: Apply a pad over the cleaned wound. Starting at the midabdomen, wrap gauze up the left side to the back and down the right side of the abdomen. Then run the gauze through the legs, staying to the left side of the tail. **Top right:** Circle the trunk by going down the right side and up the left side. Then bring the gauze over to the right side of the tail and through the legs to the left flank. Repeat this crisscross pattern at least 2 times. **Bottom:** Cover the gauze with adhesive tape, catching some fur on the edges and applying in the same crisscross pattern as the gauze. Your dog should be able to walk, urinate and defecate normally with the bandage on. If you have a male dog, you may have to cut an opening in the bandage for your dog's penis.

Foreleg/Hind leg

For any wound of the leg when you don't suspect a fracture, see Figure 4-12.

Paw

For wounds on the paw or foot, see Figure 4-13.

Tail

For wounds on the tail, see Figure 4-14.

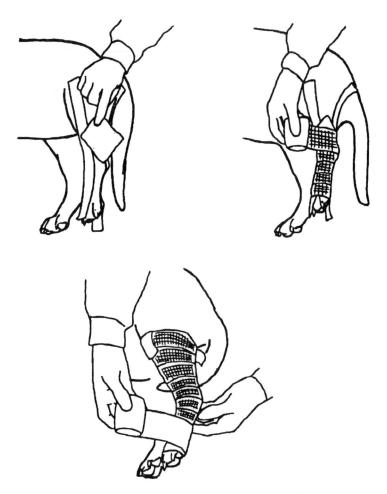

Figure 4-12: Top left: Place a pad over the cleaned wound. Place two strips of adhesive tape along the front and the back surfaces of the leg, extending a few inches above and below the wound. Place the strips so you avoid the wound, even if that means using only one strip. **Top right:** Gauze is wrapped around the leg (starting at the lower end), with evenly applied pressure, leaving one inch of adhesive tape exposed at the top and bottom. **Bottom:** Turn the exposed strips of adhesive tape onto the gauze so that the sticky side is up. Wrap adhesive tape in the same manner as the gauze, catching some fur at the edges. For full leg bandages, leave several toes visible so that you can check to see if the bandage is on too tightly. A bandage that is too tight will result in swollen, blue or cold toes. You should be able to insert easily two fingers between the bandage and the skin.

Elizabethan Collar

No matter how securely you apply a bandage, chances are that your dog will be able to remove it if given enough time. The use of an Elizabethan collar will slow your dog down considerably and should

112

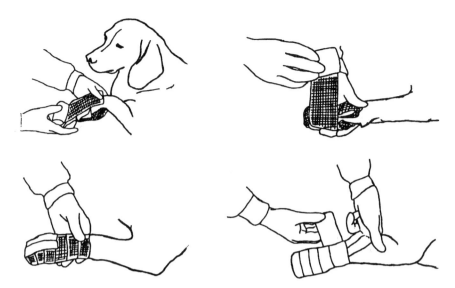

Figure 4-13: Top left: Place a pad over the cleaned wound. Use gauze folded back upon itself to cover the very bottom of the paw. **Top right:** With even pressure, wrap gauze around the paw from the bottom up to cover the layers of folded gauze. **Bottom left:** Cover the bottom of the paw with strips of adhesive tape. **Bottom right:** Wrap the adhesive tape around the foot in the same manner as the gauze. To secure the bandage, catch some fur on the top edge.

prevent her from bothering the bandages altogether. Elizabethan collars can be used to protect head bandages as well as bandages anywhere else on the body.

Your veterinarian can supply you with an Elizabethan collar for your dog. However, if you need one in an emergency (e.g., penetrating foreign object in the eye), you can easily make one as follows:

- Measure the diameter of your dog's body at the widest point (usually this will be from shoulder to shoulder).
- Cut a circular piece of cardboard half again as large as the measured diameter. Use light cardboard (for example from a gift box), if possible. If not, use the thinnest box cardboard you can find.
- Cut a hole in the center large enough to fit your dog's neck plus two fingers.
- Cut the collar on one side, from the center hole to the outer edge. Fit your dog's head into it and then tape over the cut with masking or adhesive tape (see Figure 4-15).

Stay with your dog after you put on the collar and watch the reaction. If your dog doesn't seem to adjust after a short time, especially if she becomes very nervous and madly tries to tear it off, you should remove

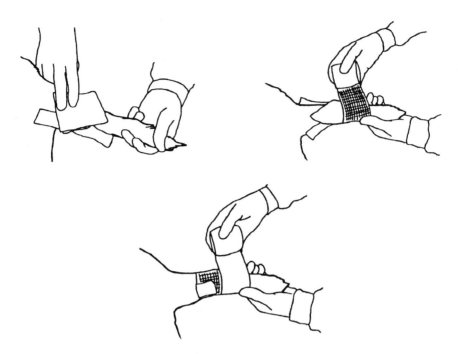

Figure 4-14: Top left: Place a pad over the cleaned wound. Place two strips of adhesive tape on the tail, avoiding the wound. Extend the tape two inches above and two inches below the wound. **Top right:** Wrap the gauze with even pressure around the tail, starting at the bottom and leaving one inch of tape exposed at the top and bottom. **Bottom:** Turn the exposed adhesive strips back onto the gauze and wrap adhesive tape around the tail, starting at the end of the reflected strip and at the bottom of the tail.

the collar. If you decide to leave the collar on, make sure that your dog can eat and drink normally while wearing it.

SECTION 3: FRACTURES

Fractures usually occur when your dog has been hit by a car, or has been subjected to some other form of severe trauma, such as falling or jumping from a high location. In this section, I will describe and illustrate two major classifications of fractures and then discuss the signs and first aid for three types of fractures: spinal, pelvic and leg.

Classification of Fractures

Open vs. Closed: An open fracture has a break in the skin caused by the bone whereas a closed fracture has no break in the skin (see Figure 4-16 [Top]).

114

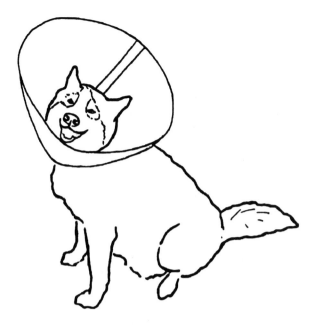

Figure 4-15: Elizabethan collar.

Simple vs. Comminuted: A simple fracture involves a bone broken into two pieces whereas a comminuted fracture has bone broken into more than two pieces (see Figure 4-16 [Bottom]).

General Signs and First Aid

Although the signs of a fracture will very much depend on its type, severity and location (see below), you may see the following signs with any type of fracture:

- Swelling
- Hot or cold skin temperature
- Bluish color to the skin

When considering first aid for fractures, it is important to remember that if your dog just suffered a severe trauma, such as being hit by a car, there may be other more serious problems (such as shock, bleeding or difficulty breathing) which need to be treated before the fracture (see Chapter 1, Section 1, Triage). The signs and first aid for specific fractures are given below.

115

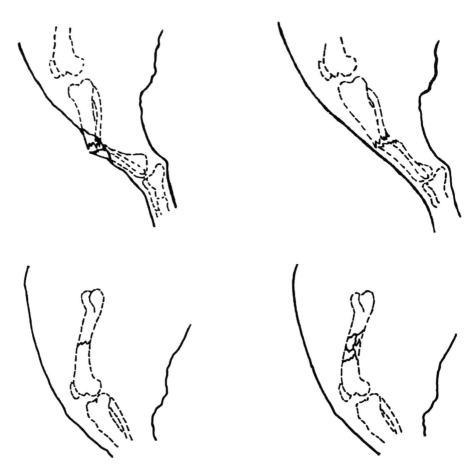

Figure 4-16: Top left: Open fracture. **Top right:** Closed fracture. **Bottom left:** Simple fracture. **Bottom right:** Comminuted fracture.

Spinal Fractures

The signs seen with spinal cord injuries will greatly depend on which part of the spinal cord is injured. In general, the signs are:

- Paralysis (inability to move or feel pain) in legs or tail
- Weakness in the legs

First Aid

- The first aid for spinal fractures is proper transport so as not to increase injury to the spinal cord (see Chapter 1, Section 2, Transporting a Dog with Spinal Cord Injuries, and Figures 1-12 and 1-13).

116

Pelvic Fractures

A dog with a pelvic fracture will be able to move her front legs normally but will be either unable to move her back legs or will try to stand up only to have her back legs immediately go out sideways.

First Aid

- If your dog is unable to move her back legs, treat just as you would a spinal fracture.
- If your dog attempts to stand up, you can help her to stay up by using adhesive tape hobbles (see Figure 4-17).

Leg Fractures

The major sign of a leg fracture is that your dog will not want to bear weight on the injured leg, although you should keep in mind that many dogs do not know this rule. If your dog is limping on one leg, it

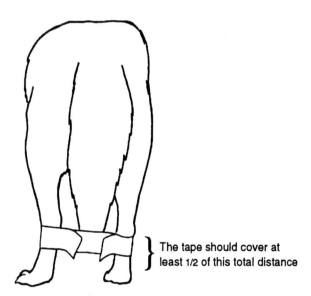

} The tape should cover at least 1/2 of this total distance

Figure 4-17: Adhesive tape hobbles. Using a wide adhesive tape, make a stirrup just below the ankle, leaving an edge of about 3 inches. Fold a small bit of the edge onto itself so you have a nonsticky tab which is easy to remove. Unwind more tape and make a stirrup on the other side, with the legs being about the same distance apart as the hips. Again, leave an edge and make a tab.

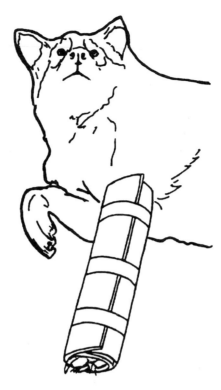

Figure 4-18: To make a temporary splint with newspaper or magazine, roll the paper around the entire leg and fasten with tape.

doesn't necessarily mean that she has a fractured leg and if she walks on her leg, it doesn't mean that the leg is not broken.

First Aid

- If you suspect a leg fracture, apply a temporary splint before moving your dog.
- You may use magazines, rolled newspapers, towels or a heavily padded bandage as a temporary splint. For a rolled newspaper splint, see Figure 4-18.
- For the best stability, the splint should cover the joint above and the joint below the suspected fracture.
- A heavily padded bandage provides the best support for a leg fracture (see Figure 4-19). If the fracture is open, apply a pad over the unwashed wound. *Do not* put ointment on the pad.

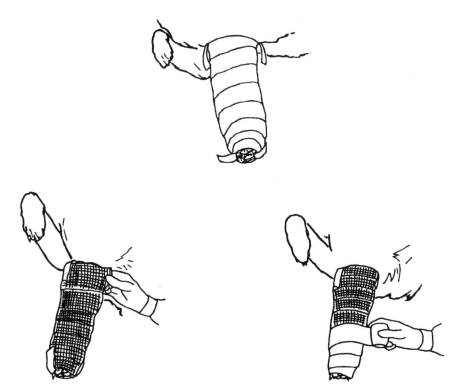

Figure 4-19: Top: To make a temporary splint with a padded bandage, absorbent cotton or a clean towel is rolled tightly around the limb after adhesive tape strips have been applied, as in Figure 4-12. Start wrapping the cotton or towel at the paw and move up. Leave one to two toes visible so that you can check to see if the bandage has been put on too tightly (swollen, blue or cold toes). **Bottom left:** Roll the gauze tightly down on the towels, starting at the paw and working up to the whole length of the leg. The strips of adhesive tape are then turned back so that the sticky side is up. **Bottom right:** The adhesive tape is applied with tension over the gauze, starting at the paw and working up. Remember to leave several toes visible.

- If no splinting supplies are available, splint the broken hind leg to the unbroken hind leg, using handkerchiefs or short pieces of gauze. *Do not* put the ties around the areas which you suspect are fractured.
- After the fracture is immobilized, check your dog from head-to-toe, as she may have suffered other injuries of which you are unaware.
- When your dog has a fracture:
  —*Never* try to manipulate the bones back into their normal place.
  —*Never* wash out fractures.

—*Never* move a dog with a leg fracture without first applying a temporary splint.

SECTION 4: DISLOCATIONS, SPRAINS AND STRAINS

Dislocations, sprains and strains may all produce the same general signs as fractures, and because of this they are usually treated in the same manner until a fracture is ruled out.

A *dislocation* occurs when a bone pops out of its joint, usually due to severe trauma. *Sprains* are torn or stretched *ligaments, tendons* and *blood vessels* around joints and are also caused by severe trauma. *Strains* are torn or stretched *muscles* around joints and are uncommon in dogs. They are caused by sudden physical exertion.

All of these conditions may produce the following signs:

- Painful joints
- Swollen joints
- Discoloration
- Limping

First Aid

- If your dog is limping, apply a temporary splint.
- If your dog is not limping and the trauma occurred within the past few hours, confine your dog and apply cool compresses to the joint. If the trauma occurred more than 24 hours ago, apply warm compresses.
- In either situation, have your veterinarian examine your dog soon to ascertain the true nature of the problem.

SUMMARY

Since wounds occur to nearly all dogs at some point in their lives, you should know how to dress a wound and apply a proper bandage. In severe trauma, such as occurs in auto accidents and falls, wounds may be complicated by fractures, dislocations and sprains. Recognizing the relevant signs, you can transport your dog in a way which will minimize the pain and complications due to the fracture.

5

Cases of
Emergency Situations:
Problem Sets

THE FOLLOWING CASES are taken from real life emergency situations. Read them through carefully and then decide what you would do. The answers are given in Appendix 3.

CASE 1:

You and your Labrador Retriever, Rufus, are traveling by car to visit your favorite uncle. You are on an interstate highway when you decide to stretch at the next rest stop and play a game of Frisbee with Rufus.

You throw the Frisbee to Rufus, but the wind catches it and takes it toward the ramp leading off the highway. Rufus dashes to catch the Frisbee, oblivious of the large truck just entering the ramp. Before you can call him back, Rufus has been hit by the truck. You find him with a large bleeding wound on his back right leg, unable to get up.

CASE 2:

Your Dachshund, Fritz, is very protective, not only of you but also of your fenced-in yard. One day, the neighbors' German Shepherd jumps the fence looking for some food.

Your dog tries to attack the Shepherd but gets attacked instead. Fritz suffers puncture wounds to the chest and abdomen in addition to a large laceration on his foreleg. He is breathing with difficulty.

CASE 3:

You own a young Standard Schnauzer, Leaping Lorelei, who loves to climb and jump fences. You install a 5 foot fence around your pool hoping this will keep Lorelei away from the pool.

It is a hot day and you must leave to do some short errands. You decide to leave Lorelei at home. You come home a short while later to find your dog struggling wildly in the water at the very edge of the pool. By the time you get to Lorelei, she has stopped struggling, is not breathing and has no pulse.

CASE 4:

You own a large, mixed-breed dog named Herbie. He loves to run, especially around in circles. He will run anytime, including after he has eaten his dinner. One day, you come home to find Herbie seemingly asleep in his doghouse. On closer inspection, you determine that Herbie is in shock with one side of his abdomen expanded and with froth near his mouth.

CASE 5:

Your Beagle puppy, Corky, loves to bite cords. You have puppy-proofed your home so Corky has not been able to discover the marvels of electricity on his own.

Your sister comes to visit for the weekend and accidently leaves her hair dryer plugged in. Your sister finds him later in the day, unresponsive with burns around his mouth and the chewed cord of the hair dryer in his mouth. Before you examine him, you unplug the hair dryer. You find his breathing has stopped and he has no pulse.

CASE 6:

You have to run an errand on a day when the outdoor temperature is over 100°F. You must take your new puppy, Lily, with you so you park in the shade and leave your window down for a little air.

You meet an old friend while doing your errand and by the time you get back, thirty minutes have gone by. Your car is no longer in the shade and Lily has collapsed in the backseat. You evaluate her and find she feels extremely hot and is not breathing but has a pulse.

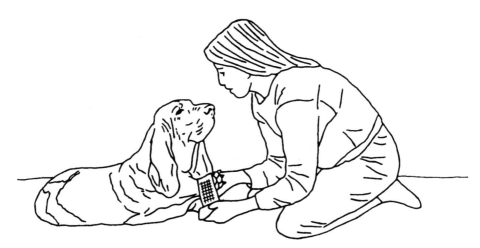
Immediate attention is the best treatment when emergencies do occur.

APPENDIX 1

How to Prevent Emergencies

CALL YOUR VETERINARIAN

In any emergency, even when you have already provided first aid, notify your veterinarian and have your dog examined. Even with minor accidents, you might have overlooked serious problems.

ELECTRICAL HAZARDS

All electrical wires should be safely stored away or at least out of sight of your dog. Out of boredom or playfulness, your dog may chew on the wires and get a serious burn in the mouth. Always remember to unplug the cord before giving first aid.

EXAMINATIONS

Make sure your dog is examined once a year by your veterinarian. Catch problems before they start.

FOOD

Never feed your dog table food, as it is usually too high in fat. Feed commercial food or a home-made diet approved by your veterinarian. Always provide plenty of fresh water and limit exercise for about 2 hours following meals.

POISONS

Keep your cleaners, polishers, bleaches and detergents high up or under the sink in a locked cabinet. Many common household chemicals may cause your dog to become sick (Table 3-1).

Houseplants should be kept high up and out of the way of your dog. Many plants can make your dog sick and some may even cause severe illness or death (see Table 3-2).

Keep your dog's medicines, as well as your own, high up or in a locked cabinet. Never give medications to your dog without first checking with your veterinarian.

RESTRAINT

Keep your dog on a leash when outside of the house. Let him run free in large, fenced areas.

TRASH

Keep your garbage secure both inside and outside of your house.

TRAVELING

When traveling with your dog, be sure to use a carrier or kennel which is secured in your car. *Never* let your dog put his head outside of an open window, and *never* allow your dog to travel in the back of an open pickup truck.

WEATHER

In the summertime make sure your dog has access to shade, fresh air and cool water. Avoid leaving your dog in your car. If you must, do so for only short periods with the window open a small amount in the shade.

In the winter, after walking your dog on to the road, be sure to wash the road salts off the dog's paws.

APPENDIX 2

Medications and Dosages

Oral medications may be given in liquid form or in pill form.

When giving liquid medicine, it might be easier to try mixing it into a little bit of your dog's favorite canned food. If this doesn't work, use a plastic medicine dropper. These droppers are calibrated in teaspoons and can be purchased in a pharmacy. Give the medicine in an even movement with the dropper pointed toward the base of the tongue, not up at the roof of the mouth (see Figure A-1 [Left]).

When giving a pill, first try to hide it inside of a little bit of canned food or peanut butter, then offer it to your dog. If this doesn't work, pill your dog as shown in Figure A-1 [Right], holding the dog's mouth open and throwing the pill toward the back. To make it easier for your dog to swallow the pill, smear the pill with a small amount of honey. Once you have thrown the pill into your dog's mouth, close his mouth and rub the throat to encourage the dog to swallow.

Never give oral medication to a dog who is vomiting, unconscious, choking or gagging. Always check with your veterinarian before giving your dog any medications.

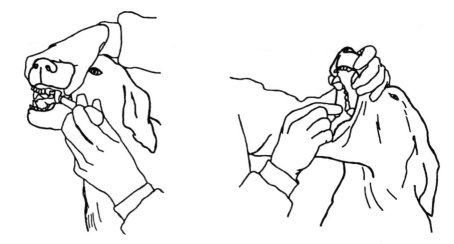

Figure A-1: Left: To give liquid medication with a medicine dropper, hold the upper jaw with one hand, while the other hand holds the medicine dropper. Point the dropper toward the bottom of the mouth and give the medicine slowly and evenly. **Right:** To give your dog a pill, hold the upper jaw with one hand while the other hand holds the lower jaw open and throws the pill toward the back of the mouth.

ANTIBIOTIC OINTMENT

- Reduces the chance of infection if used on a pad as part of a bandage (see Chapter 4, Section 2).
- Use Neosporin® or Bacitracin.

ASPIRIN

- Use buffered or enteric-coated aspirin only.
- Relieves pain, reduces fever and inflammation.
- Dosage: 5.5 mg/lb, twice per day. (For example, a 15 pound dog would get ¼ adult aspirin or 1 baby aspirin twice per day; a 30 pound dog would get ½ adult aspirin twice per day; and a 60 pound dog would get 1 adult aspirin twice per day.) Give aspirin with food to reduce stomach irritation.

ACTIVATED CHARCOAL POWDER

- Absorbs small amounts of poison after vomiting has occurred.
- Dosage: For a dog under 25 pounds, give 1 teaspoon mixed to a

slurry with water once. For a dog over 25 pounds, give 2 teaspoons mixed to slurry with water once.

HYDROGEN PEROXIDE (3%)

- Induces vomiting.
- Dosage: 1 to 2 teaspoons by mouth every 15 minutes until vomiting starts.

SYRUP OF IPECAC

- Induces vomiting.
- Dosage: Give 2 to 3 teaspoons one time.

VEGETABLE OIL, MINERAL OIL

- Coats the intestine and helps pass poisons through the gastrointestinal tract.
- Dosage: For a dog under 25 pounds, give 1 to 2 teaspoons once by mouth. For a dog over 25 pounds, give 1 to 2 tablespoons once by mouth.

APPENDIX 3

Answers to Cases

CASE 1:

Before attending to the wound on Rufus's leg, you should quickly take his temperature, pulse and respiration rate. You should also look at his gums to check the capillary refill time and color.

If these parameters indicate shock, then you should cover Rufus with a towel or blanket and keep him still. If Rufus isn't in shock, he might well be later, so you should check him again after you have tended to the wound.

To stop the bleeding on his back right leg, first try pressure directly on the wound. If this doesn't work and you can get to this location without too much manipulation of the leg, try pressing on the femoral artery (see Figure 1-42). *Moving the leg around too much might increase the pain and swelling if the leg is fractured.* For the same reason, do not elevate the leg. You should suspect that Rufus probably has a fractured leg and may have suffered other fractures (pelvis, spine) because of his inability to stand up and because his wounded leg is so painful.

At this point, you should apply a temporary splint to the injured leg, using, for example, a newspaper or magazine and tape. Remember *not to wash* the wound if it is an open fracture. After the splint is on, check again to see if Rufus is in shock.

If you don't have a large board and people to help you, then you should pick Rufus up by putting one arm between his front legs and one arm between his back legs. You should then carry your dog by keeping his back as straight as possible. Place Rufus in your car, laying him on his side with the splint leg up. Then find a phone and call the nearest veterinarian to have Rufus's wounds and fracture treated.

CASE 2:

Although Fritz has suffered many wounds, his most serious problem is breathing. The first step is to open his mouth and make sure that the airway is not obstructed.

If you have help, have the other person drive you and Fritz to your veterinarian while you continue with first aid. You should then take your dog's respiration rate, pulse and temperature, in addition to the capillary refill time and mucous membrane color. These parameters will probably tell you that Fritz is in shock. To treat the shock, cover Fritz with a light blanket and keep him still.

Next you should take care of the wounds. Since Fritz's breathing difficulties may be due to an open chest wound, be sure *not to wash the wound* but apply a wet pad dressing immediately after your dog exhales. Then take care of the abdominal wounds and the laceration.

As soon as these are covered, call your veterinarian if you haven't already done so. Continue to monitor Fritz until he can be treated.

CASE 3:

Your first concern in a case such as this is to remove as much water as you can from your dog's lungs. The best way to do this is first to open the airway. Then hold Lorelei upside down by wrapping your arms around her lower abdomen and sway back and forth for 30 seconds.

If someone is present who can drive you, you should call your veterinarian and perform **CPR** on the way to the clinic. If you are by yourself, you should give **CPR** until Lorelei is breathing on her own and has a pulse. You will be giving 2 breaths for every 15 compressions at a rate of 80 to 100 compressions per minute. At this point, you should call your veterinarian and monitor your dog until she can be thoroughly examined.

CASE 4:

Herbie has the classic signs of bloat (gastric torsion). You must act quickly if you are to save your dog.

First, call your veterinarian and, if you have access to a car, transport Herbie to the veterinary hospital. If you do not have access to a car, have a neighbor drive you to the clinic or call a taxi. In the car, cover Herbie with a blanket to keep his body temperature from dropping further and to keep him from going deeper into shock.

CASE 5:

Corky has suffered an electric shock. In a case such as this, do not be distracted by the burns around his mouth, which may be severe. Your biggest concern must be to start **CPR** as soon as possible.

If you have access to a car and someone who can drive you, have her call your veterinarian and drive you to the veterinary hospital. Meanwhile, you can start **CPR** at home and continue in the car.

If it is not possible for you to get to your veterinarian right away, start **CPR** and continue until a pulse returns and breathing begins. For a puppy, you will be compressing both sides of the chest at a rate of at least 120 times per minute and giving a breath on every sixth compression.

CASE 6:

Your puppy, Lily, has suffered heat stroke. Obviously, you must start giving artificial respirations, but before doing this, take a second to carry Lily into a shady area where there is fresh air.

Now you can start artificial respirations at a rate of *20 to 25 breaths per minute*. If you have help and have access to a car, you can continue breathing for your puppy while someone takes you to the closest emergency clinic or veterinary hospital. If you are by yourself, continue artificial respirations, stopping to check the pulse every minute or so.

Once her breathing has returned, call your veterinarian. Continue to monitor your puppy until she can be examined.

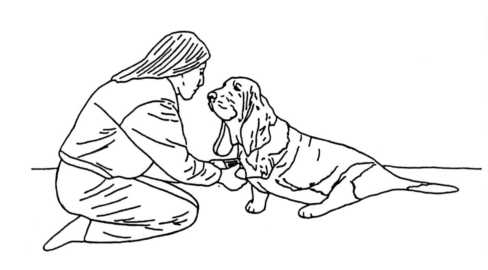

Bibliography

American Red Cross. *American Red Cross Standard First Aid Workbook.* American National Red Cross, 1988.

Behler, John L. and F. Wayne King. *The Audubon Society Field Guide to North American Reptiles and Amphibians.* New York: Alfred A. Knopf, 1979.

Ettinger, Stephen J., ed. *Textbook of Veterinary Internal Medicine. Diseases of the Dog and Cat,* 2nd ed. Vols. 1 and 2. Philadelphia: W. B. Saunders Co., 1983.

Fowler, Murray E. *Plant Poisoning in Small Companion Animals.* Saint Louis: Ralston Purina, Co., 1980.

Fraser, Clarence M., ed. *The Merck Veterinary Manual,* 6th ed. Rahway: Merck & Co., 1986.

Kirk, Robert W., ed. *Current Veterinary Therapy, VIII.* Philadelphia: W. B. Saunders Co., 1983.

Kirk, Robert W. and Stephen I. Bistner. *Handbook of Veterinary Procedures and Emergency Treatment.* Philadelphia: W. B. Saunders Co., 1981.

Knecht, Charles D. *Fundamental Techniques in Veterinary Surgery.* Philadelphia: W. B. Saunders Co., 1981.

Muller, George H. *Small Animal Dermatology.* Philadelphia: W. B. Saunders Co., 1983.

Proceedings of the Second International Veterinary Emergency and Critical Care Symposium. September 16–19, 1990. San Antonio: Pro-Visions Pet Specialty Enterprises, 1990.

Proceedings of the Third International Veterinary Emergency and Critical Care Symposium. September 20–23, 1992. San Antonio: Pro-Visions Canine Nutrition Management, 1992.

Stamp, Gary L., ed. *Veterinary Clinics of North America: Small Animal Practice,* Vol. 19, No. 6, Philadelphia: W. B. Saunders Co., 1989.

Zaslow, Ira M., ed. *Veterinary Trauma and Critical Care*. Philadelphia: Lea & Febiger, 1984.

Glossary

Abrasion—a type of wound which occurs when the skin is scraped by a hard surface.

Airway—the path by which air enters the body and flows to and from the lungs.

Ambulatory—able to walk.

Amputation—the severance of a body part, usually a leg, from the rest of the body.

Anaphylactic shock—a type of allergic reaction which occurs within a few minutes.

Anemic—a reduction in the number of red blood cells or hemoglobin in the blood, causing weakness.

Artificial respiration—a type of rescue breathing where air is forced from the mouth of the rescuer into the nose and lungs of the victim.

Avulsion—a tearing of a body part from the rest of the body without complete separation.

Bloat—the filling of the stomach with gas. Bloat may lead to gastric torsion.

Capillary refill time—the time it takes the tiny blood vessels under the skin to refill once they have been emptied by manual pressure.

Cardiopulmonary failure—an absence of normal heart and lung function.

Cardiopulmonary resuscitation—a technique which combines artificial respiration and chest compressions in cases where the heart and lungs cease to function.

Circulation—the flow of blood through the body. Circulation may be assessed by checking the pulse, color of the gums and capillary refill time.

Closed fracture—a broken bone not accompanied by a break in the skin.

Closed wound—a wound where the skin is not broken; also known as a bruise or contusion.

Coma—a complete loss of consciousness with no response to pain.

Comminuted fracture—a type of fracture where the bone is broken into *more* than 2 pieces.

Cornea—the outer, visible layer of the eyeball.

Dehydration—a condition which indicates loss of body water. Dehydration is commonly caused by vomiting and diarrhea. Dehydration may lead to shock.

Dermis—the lower layer of the skin.

Dislocation—a condition which occurs when a bone comes out of its joint.

Eclampsia—muscle tremors which occur in the female dog after whelping.

Electric shock—a condition resulting from contact of the body with an exposed wire.

Elizabethan collar—a type of collar which extends outward from the neck and is designed to prevent a dog from removing a bandage, licking a wound or scratching certain areas.

Epidermis—the top layer of the skin.

Epilepsy—a disorder of the central nervous system, characterized by seizures.

Finger sweep—a technique used to check the mouth of a choking dog.

Foreign body—an object which may become lodged in the airway causing blockage.

Frostbite—the freezing of small areas of the body due to exposure to the cold.

Full thickness burn—a burn which involves the entire thickness of the skin; also known as a third degree burn.

Gastric torsion—a state in which a gas-filled stomach twists upon itself, cuts off the blood supply leading to shock and death.

Glaucoma—a condition resulting from increased pressure within the eye.

Grand mal seizure—a type of generalized seizure characterized by the presence of convulsions. (See Epilepsy).

Head-to-toe exam—an evaluation of the major body systems to check for problems which are not obvious.

Heat stroke—an internal body temperature of 105 degrees or higher usually resulting from confinement or overexposure in hot weather.

Heimlich-like maneuver—an abdominal thrust performed just below the sternum or rib cage to remove a foreign object lodged in the airway.

Hematoma—a swelling which contains blood. Usually found on the ear.

Hemorrhage—severe bleeding.

Hives—a type of allergic reaction which takes about 20 minutes to develop and involves redness and swelling in the eyes and mouth.

Hobbles—a stirrup fastened just below the ankles which keeps the legs together and the animal standing.

Hypersensitive—an increased ability to show allergic symptoms when in contact with certain substances, such as specific foods or drugs.

Hypothermia—generalized body chilling due to exposure to the cold.

Incision—a type of wound which results from being cut by a sharp object with smooth, straight edges.

Infection—the condition of a wound which becomes invaded by microorganisms. The major signs seen are pain, redness, swelling and heat. Also an internal condition sometimes characterized by anemia or changes in the white blood cell count.

Insidious condition—a problem which develops gradually and without readily visible signs.

Insulin—a substance used to lower blood sugar in the treatment of diabetes.

Intussusception—a condition which occurs when one part of the intestine pushes into the inside of another part.

Laceration—a type of wound which occurs when the skin is cut by an object with sharp irregular edges.

Low grade fever—an internal body temperature of 1 to 2 degrees above normal.

Muzzle—a restraining device covering the mouth of the dog to prevent biting. Also, the dog's foreface.

Obstruction—blockage of the airway or any part of the gastrointestinal tract.

Open fracture—a broken bone accompanied by a break in the skin.

Open wound—a type of wound in which the skin is broken.

Paralysis—the inability to move or feel pain.

Partial thickness burn—a type of burn which involves the entire epidermis and part of the dermis; also known as a second degree burn.

Petit mal seizure—a type of generalized seizure in which no convulsions occur. (See Epilepsy.)

Pressure point—a point where hand pressure is applied to the main artery supplying the bleeding area.

Prolapse—a condition which occurs when a body part slips out of its normal location, e.g., eye or rectum.

Pulse—the throbbing of the heartbeat as felt in the major arteries. The pulse is commonly taken by lightly pressing in the groin, which is the location of the femoral artery.

Puncture wound—a type of wound which is caused by a pointed object, such as a tooth.

Pupil size—the size of the opening at the center of the colored portion of the eye.

Rectum—the end of the gastrointestinal tract, which opens out to the anus.

Respiration rate—the number of breaths taken per minute.

Responsive—the ability to react to a number of actions, such as calling, clapping or touching.

Restraint—a technique of holding or applying a muzzle which allows the rescuer to give first aid safely.

Retinal detachment—the separation of the innermost part of the eye from its outer covering. This usually occurs as a result of severe trauma.

Shock—a condition resulting from circulatory system failure. It must be treated immediately because it can quickly lead to unconsciousness and death.

Simple fracture—a type of fracture where the bone is broken into no more than two pieces.

Skin elasticity—the ability of the skin to stretch.

Splint—a rigid bandage used to keep movement to a minimum in cases of dislocations and fractures.

Sprain—a condition which results from torn or stretched ligaments, tendons and blood vessels around joints.

Stabilized—a condition which is not changing and one in which the victim is not in immediate danger of dying.

Sternum—breastbone; the site at which chest compressions are done in large dogs.

Strain—a condition which results from torn or stretched muscles around joints.

Superficial burn—a burn which involves only the epidermis; also known as a first degree burn.

Support—being able to transport a dog so the spinal column stays straight.

Tetanus—a disease caused by *Clostridium tetani* bacteria growing in puncture wounds.

Tourniquet—a very constrictive band which is applied as a last resort to stop severe bleeding.

Tracheal collapse—a condition which occurs when the tissues supporting the airway are too soft or the airway itself is too small to remain open.

Transport—a technique of moving a dog safely without causing further injury.

Triage—a technique which involves making a quick assessment of the major problems and sorting these problems from most severe to least severe.

Umbilicus—navel; the site where the umbilical cord was attached to the placenta; located midabdominally.

Urethra—the tube which connects the bladder to the external opening.

Urinary tract blockage—a condition which occurs when the urethra becomes obstructed.

Urolith—a small stone composed of mineral salts which forms in the urinary tract and may cause blockage.

Index